Sports Medicine, Performance Enhancement and Doping

Tracing the history of sports medicine from the ancient world through to the present day, this book shines new light on the embedded relationship between physicians, performance enhancement and doping in elite sport.

Combining historical and sociological analysis, this book shows how sports medicine, as it developed in the late nineteenth and twentieth centuries, became increasingly disengaged from its origins in preventive medicine to become closely linked with elite-level competitive sport. This book demonstrates how this link between sports medicine and elite competitive sport drew sports physicians into the search for enhanced performance so that by the second half of the twentieth century performance enhancement had become an essential raison d'être of sports medicine practitioners. It examines how this search for enhanced performance has often led sports physicians to play a prominent role in the development and provision of performance-enhancing drugs, and looks in depth at the case study of France and professional cycling, scene of some of the most high-profile and consequential doping cases of all time.

This book is fascinating reading for anybody with an interest in sport history, the history of medicine, medical ethics, the ethics of sport, sport and society, or science and society.

Ivan Waddington is Visiting Professor at the University of Chester, UK. His books include *Sport, Health and Drugs* (E & F N Spon, 2000), *Drugs in Sport* (BMJ Books, 2002), *An Introduction to Drugs in Sport* (with Andy Smith, Routledge, 2009), *Pain and Injury in Sport* (with Sigmund Loland and Berit Skirstad, Routledge, 2006), and he was co-editor (with Verner Møller and John Hoberman) of the *Routledge Handbook of Drugs and Sport* (Routledge, 2015). His work has been translated into French, German, Italian, Spanish, Flemish and Japanese.

Christophe Brissonneau is a researcher in the Department of Sports Science, University of Paris Cité, France. He has authored many journal articles on the subject of doping in sport, and his books include *Doping in Elite Sport: Voices of French Sportspeople and Their Doctors, 1950 2000* (with Jeffrey Montez de Oca, Routledge, 2018), *L'Epreuve du Dopage* (O. Aubel F. Ohl, PUF, 2008). He supervised a group of experts for the European Parliament study *Doping in Professional Sport* (2008).

Sports Medicine, Performance Enhancement and Doping

A Critical History

Ivan Waddington and Christophe Brissonneau

Routledge
Taylor & Francis Group
LONDON AND NEW YORK

First published 2025
by Routledge
4 Park Square, Milton Park, Abingdon, Oxon OX14 4RN

and by Routledge
605 Third Avenue, New York, NY 10158

Routledge is an imprint of the Taylor & Francis Group, an informa business

British Library Cataloguing-in-Publication Data
A catalogue record for this book is available from the British Library

ISBN: 978-1-032-91562-3 (hbk)
ISBN: 978-1-032-91568-5 (pbk)
ISBN: 978-1-003-56392-1 (ebk)

DOI: 10.4324/9781003563921

Typeset in Times New Roman
by Deanta Global Publishing Services, Chennai, India

Ivan dedicates this book to his wife Sue

Christophe dedicates this book to Sidonie, Mewenn and Gwenaëlle

Contents

Tables

Contributor

Jeffrey Montez de Oca is Professor of Sociology and Founding Director of the Center for the Critical Studies of Sport in the University of Colorado. His research has focused on college football, media, NFL marketing and outdoor sports.

Introduction

Understanding the development of sports medicine

During the last four decades or so there have been numerous scandals involving drug use in elite sport. Among these, one might perhaps highlight the following as being of particular significance: the positive drug test of Canadian sprinter Ben Johnson at the 1988 Seoul Olympic Games; the revelations by French police concerning widespread drug use in the 1998 Tour de France; the investigation by the United States Anti-Doping Agency (USADA) which, in 2012, revealed systematic drug use over many years by seven times Tour de France winner, Lance Armstrong, and other riders within Armstrong's US Postal Service and Discovery Channel cycling teams; and, most recently, evidence of the widespread, state-sponsored drug use by Russian athletes.

Not only did all these scandals receive massive media coverage but they were also significant for other reasons. Johnson's positive test at the Seoul Olympics led to the establishment by the Canadian Government of the Dubin Commission, whose report provided the first systematically collected, reliable and detailed body of evidence about the social organisation of drug use in elite sport (Dubin, 1990). The police investigation into drug use in the 1998 Tour de France not only resulted in a number of legal trials and convictions which, in a comparable fashion to the Dubin Report, revealed in great detail the organisation of drug use in professional cycling (Waddington, 2000; Waddington and Smith, 2009) but also acted as a catalyst for the establishment of the World Anti-Doping Agency (WADA) at the Lausanne Conference in 1999 (Hanstad, Smith and Waddington, 2008). USADA's investigation of Armstrong (USADA, 2012) and the McLaren investigation into the state-sponsored drugs programme in Russia (McLaren, 2016a, 2016b) both provided further detailed analyses of the social organisation of doping networks. In addition, both the USADA investigation of Armstrong, who had been regularly tested for drugs throughout his career but had never been sanctioned on the basis of a failed test, and, perhaps even more so, the fact that the Russian state-sponsored drugs programme, involving more than a thousand athletes in more than thirty sports, was revealed not as a result of drug testing but as a consequence of the actions of a whistleblower within the drugs programme, clearly highlighted the ineffectiveness of WADA's traditional reliance on biological testing as the basis of its anti-doping policy (Waddington, 2019, Waddington and Møller, 2019).

These scandals differed from each other in a variety of ways. The Dubin Commission focused mainly on drug use in Canadian sport, while the primary

DOI: 10.4324/9781003563921-1

focus of the USADA investigation was the American cycling teams in which Armstrong had been involved. The central focus of the investigation by French police into drug use in the Tour de France was of course professional cycling in France, though cyclists and team officials from several other nations were also involved. The revelations about drug use in Russia concerned a major eastern European superpower, in both sporting and non-sporting terms. And while the French and American scandals focused on professional cycling, the Canadian and Russian cases both involved drug use in a wide variety of Olympic sports.

However, despite these differences, all these cases have two important characteristics in common. The first of these is that none of them supported the common stereotype of the drug-using athlete – a stereotype which, it might be added, anti-doping organisations have often sought to convey and which has long formed a cornerstone of many aspects of anti-doping policy: the highly individualised conception of the drug-using athlete as an asocial, isolated, lone 'bad apple', working alone (Waddington, 2019; Waddington and Møller, 2019). In marked contrast to this misleading stereotype, the investigations into all these cases revealed that drug-using athletes almost never work alone; rather, they are typically involved in what has been called a 'doping network' (Waddington, 2000: 159), that is a network of relationships involving a variety of people, sometimes in several countries, occupying different positions within sport, in the supply, use and monitoring of the drugs, and in the concealment of their use.

The second characteristic which all these cases have in common is that central to the doping network in each case were practitioners of sports medicine, often team doctors. Thus the Dubin Commission revealed not only that Dr Jamie Astaphan had supplied Ben Johnson with drugs and monitored his drug use, but also that Dr Astaphan was widely regarded within sport as an expert on the use of performance-enhancing drugs and that he had an international clientele of elite athletes from many countries in North America, Europe and Africa. Dubin also revealed the existence of a network of doctors across North America who prescribed performance-enhancing drugs for athletes. The police investigation into drug use at the 1998 Tour de France (which is the basis of a major case study in Chapter 10) revealed that team doctors were central to the systematic organisation of drug use within teams, with the doctors of three leading teams being charged under the 1989 Anti-Drug Act in France, which prohibited 'the administration, enticement to use or facilitation of employment of substances or doping procedures during competitions or sporting events' (Waddington, 2000: 156–159). Similarly, the USADA investigation generated 'more than enough evidence to proceed with charges' not only against Armstrong, but also against three former team doctors, Pedro Celaya, Luis Garcia del Moral and, most significantly, Professor Michele Ferrari (USADA, 2012: 4). And as the McLaren Report made clear, those who ran the Russian state-sponsored drugs programme were 'assisted ... by various informed medical personnel' (McLaren, 2016a: 8); it might be noted that in this regard the Russian state-sponsored programme simply mirrored the earlier Soviet state-sponsored doping programme which, as Riordan (1991: 122–123, emphasis in original) has noted, 'was organised *at the top* and involved parts of the sports medical establishment'.

In terms of the involvement of practitioners of sports medicine, these examples are not unusual. In Italy, one could point to the work of Francesco Conconi, described by Paoli (2019: 83) as 'the father of Italian "doping physicians"'. Paoli notes that, in Germany, 'Conconi's pendant was represented by the work of Armin Klümper and Joseph Keul, two former sports physicians at the University of Freiburg which, in the 1970s and 1980s, treated up to 80-90% of the West German elite athletes'. She notes that they used a variety of techniques – including the use of 'doping products' – to make them competitive with athletes from East Germany and other Soviet bloc countries which had centralised systems of 'state doping' (Paoli, 2019: 84). In Spain in 2006, a police investigation, codenamed Operación Puerto, uncovered an extensive 'blood doping' network for elite athletes operating out of the Madrid clinic of Dr Eufemiano Fuentes (Waddington and Smith, 2009: 81). More recently, a coordinated investigation by the German and Austrian police, codenamed Operation Aderlass ('bloodletting' in English) revealed a blood doping scheme for athletes which had been operated by Dr Mark Schmidt from 2011 until his arrest in 2019. Schmidt had formerly been the team doctor at two professional cycling teams, Gerolsteiner and Milram, and his clients included athletes who had competed at the 2014 and 2018 Winter Olympics, the 2016 Summer Olympics and the 2018 Tour de France (*Cycling News*, 12 January 2021). As Hoberman (2002: 207) has noted, 'the doping of athletes by sports physicians is more than a fringe phenomenon'. Indeed, it is difficult to think of any major drugs scandal in modern sport in which practitioners of sports medicine have not been centrally involved.

These data do not fit easily with the public image of practitioners of sports medicine as a group of practitioners who provide specialised medical support to our sporting heroes, returning them to play as soon as possible following injury, as well as playing an active role in developing anti-doping policies. In relation to the latter, some British scholars have pointed to what they describe as the 'greatest untold story' of the role of British doctors in the development of doping tests and anti-doping policies (Dimeo, 2007: 14; Heggie, 2011: 8). Certainly it is the case that some sports physicians have played a prominent role in the development of anti-doping policies, but an even greater untold story – at least in terms of public awareness – is that practitioners of sports medicine have also played a leading role in the development, supply and dissemination of performance-enhancing drugs and techniques and in monitoring their use by athletes; put succinctly, sports medicine 'has been one of the major contexts within which performance-enhancing drugs have been developed and used' (Waddington, 1996: 186).

However, the involvement of sports physicians in the development, dissemination and use of performance-enhancing substances and techniques has been conspicuously absent from histories of sports medicine. This is, perhaps, particularly the case where histories of sports medicine have been written by 'insiders', that is by practising sports physicians whose personal involvement in, and commitment to, sports medicine appears to have prevented the development of an appropriate level of detachment in studying the history of their own discipline. Consider, for example, the case of Germany. Germany played an important part in the development of modern sports medicine, but it is also the case, as Krüger (2015: 331) has noted, that

> sports medicine in Germany is associated with various doping scandals … beginning with the Sports Medical Service in the former East Germany … [and] the West-German networks of doping doctors like those at Freiburg University, represented by such protagonists as Joseph Keul and Armin Klümper.

However, Krüger notes that while there are several published histories of sports medicine in Germany, there is no properly 'independent and critical overview' of that history, and he suggests that this is partly because 'active sports doctors and scientists wrote their own history'. In this regard, he refers to Hollmann and Tittel's *Geschichte der deutschen Sportmedizin* (2008). Both authors were leading sports physicians in Germany and he suggests that their personal involvement in the discipline has 'prevented them from writing a critical and independent history [of German sports medicine] including their dark sides in both German dictatorships and in West Germany' (Krüger, 2015: 333).

Noting that the involvement of sports physicians in doping in the former East Germany was not the only 'ugly spot in the would-be clean slate of German sports medicine', Krüger (2015: 334) adds that: 'However, the German Society for Sports Medicine and Prevention celebrated its 100th birthday in 2012 in a highly self-conscious and confident manner. No word of self-criticism was evident either at the jubilee or in various publications' which, he suggests, should be regarded 'less as serious and objective historical research, and more as "anniversary publications"'.

The same criticism may be made of Berg and König's (2002) paper on the history of German sports medicine. As Paoli (2019) has documented, Freiburg University was, for at least half a century, a major centre of doping in German sport but, despite the fact that Berg and König's paper focuses specifically on sports medicine at the University of Freiburg, it contains no mention of doping. Both Berg and Konig, it might be noted, were sports physicians at Freiburg. Examples of similarly sanitised histories of sports medicine by sports physicians in other countries are not difficult to find (e.g. Ryan, 1989; Tipton, 1997).

In marked contrast to these histories written by 'insiders', several social scientists have drawn attention to the relationship between the institutionalisation of sports medicine in its modern form and the widespread dissemination and use of drugs to enhance sporting performance since the 1960s (Waddington, 1996, 2000, 2001, 2004, 2005, 2007, 2015, 2016, 2019; Hoberman, 1992a, 2002, 2012, 2013; Brissonneau, 2015; Brissonneau and Montez de Oca, 2018; Paoli, 2019; Paoli and Donati, 2014; Krüger, 2015).

But how is it that sports medicine has developed this Janus-faced character? (Dunning and Waddington, 2003). How is it that sports physicians have not only been involved in developing and defining the concept of doping and in developing anti-doping policies, but that they have also played a prominent part in the development and use of performance-enhancing drugs? How can we understand this process of the development of sports medicine which has culminated in a situation in which practitioners of sports medicine have been involved in almost every major sporting drugs scandal in recent decades? This is the central question which we seek to answer in this book.

Theoretical orientation and key concepts

In seeking to understand the development of modern sports medicine we have drawn upon the theoretical work of several authors. Particularly important in providing an overarching framework has been the work of Norbert Elias, particularly his emphasis on the importance of understanding long-term social processes, his concept of figurations and his work on the sociology of knowledge and science.

The development of sports medicine into the form in which we know it today, that is as a specialised body of knowledge and practice within the medical profession with its own institutional structure – colleges, specialist qualifications, conferences, journals and recognised career structures – is a relatively recent process which dates from the twentieth century and, in particular, from the second half of the twentieth century. However, we cannot understand the practice of modern sports medicine if we simply examine the present-day situation. Elias (2009a: 4) emphasised the importance of understanding what he called 'long-term transformations', that is 'transformations usually encompassing not less than three generations … of the figurations formed by human beings' and he was highly critical of those sociological approaches which focus simply on the present; such approaches, he argued, involved both 'process reduction' – the reduction of social processes to static conditions – and a 'retreat to the present' (Elias, 1978a, 1987a) which, precisely because it ignores the past, can offer only a limited understanding of the present. Following Elias, it is a fundamental principle underlying this book that we cannot understand the modern structure of sports medicine without examining how that structure has developed as a long-term social process.

Accordingly, we have adopted what might be described as an 'historical' approach. However, we have used inverted commas to differentiate our approach from what might be considered a more conventional historical approach. In order to understand some of the specificities of our approach, it is necessary briefly to say something about another of Elias's key concepts, that of figuration. Elias (1978b: 261) defined a figuration as 'a structure of mutually oriented and dependent people' and he developed the concept as a means of emphasising the interdependencies between people and of overcoming a number of what he regarded as misleading and unhelpful dualisms and dichotomies within sociology, one of which was that between the individual and society (Elias, 1978a, 2009b). Elias suggested that the concept of figuration leads to an easy transition from the '*Homo clausus*' image of the human being (conceptualised in the singular) as an asocial, isolated, 'closed person', to the more adequate conceptualisation of humans (in the plural) as '*Homines aperti*', that is 'open people', bonded together with other people in various ways and whose actions and choices are constrained, to varying degrees, by those bonds with others (Elias, 1978a: 125). While fully recognising the importance of the process of individualisation in modern societies – the process as a result of which we have come to think of ourselves as individuals, separate from others – Elias emphasised, particularly in *The Society of Individuals* (1991), that the process of individualisation is itself a *social* process and he was at pains to stress that the concept of figuration 'draws attention to people's interdependencies' (Elias, 1978a: 132). Just as the concept of people's interdependencies was central to Elias's sociology, so too is it central to our approach to understanding the development of sports medicine.

But what does this mean in practice? It means that those who are looking for a history of sports medicine as the history of outstanding individual practitioners or researchers and their discoveries will be disappointed. This is not to say, of course, that some scientists are not more able, more far-sighted or more creative than others. But it is to say that the development of science cannot be understood if we focus on individual scientists or doctors, conceptualised as *Homo clausus*, as isolated individuals. The problem here has been nicely pointed out by Elias, who noted that one question which frequently arises in the work of historians of science is: 'Who was the first individual putting on record such and such a scientific idea?' He suggests:

> This type of problem undoubtedly has its place in enquiries in the development of a science, but the exaggerated value often attached to priority questions of this type among historians of science is closely connected with the unspoken assumption that in making his (sic) contribution to the growth of science each individual scientist is, as it were, wholly on his own and that it depends wholly on his own individual ingenuity in posing and solving problems.
>
> (Elias, 1972: 123)

He adds that historians of science

> often think it enough to present us with a narrative of the deeds and views of a few selected and often only of a few outstanding [scientists] … it must be enough to point to the fact that the study of the growth of scientific knowledge and especially the classification of the sequential order of the growth requires something more than the stringing together, by means of a largely arbitrary narrative, of individual ideas, selected according to largely uncharted conventions.
>
> (Elias, 1972: 123–124)

Elsewhere, he writes that, in acquiring knowledge, 'no human being is a beginning … everybody stands on the shoulders of others from whom he (sic) has learned an already acquired fund of knowledge', adding that the 'classical epistemological paradigm of a lonely individual, an isolated 'subject' fishing here and now for knowledge of the connections of 'objects' in the vastness of an unknown world, starting from scratch and all on his own, is no longer serviceable' (Elias, 2009c: 22–23).

By way of setting out a more adequate approach to understanding the development of science, Elias (1972: 130) used the example of quantum mechanics:

> I find it difficult to imagine that anybody can hope to explain or to understand the transition from classical to quantum mechanics without reference to the changes in technology that have occurred between the seventeenth and the twentieth centuries; these technological changes, in turn, cannot be understood and explained without reference to changes in the overall structure of societies where these technological and scientific changes have taken place; these changes in the overall structure of societies, again, can neither be understood nor explained without reference to the scientific changes.

Elias continually emphasised that scientific knowledge constituted a *social* fund of knowledge and, underlying everything we have written in this book is the fundamental premise which runs through all Elias's writings: that science is a *social* activity and that developments in science and medicine can only be understood as *social processes*.

The central implication of this premise is that one cannot understand the development of sports medicine, as a body of knowledge or as a form of practice, without locating practitioners of sports medicine within the figurations – the networks of relationships – in which they were involved. Moreover these figurations have changed radically over the last two hundred years. At the beginning of the nineteenth century, the interest of physicians in physical activity was limited to encouraging their patients to engage in what they saw as healthy forms of exercise and the figurations in which physicians were involved were for the most part small, local and relatively simple, consisting largely of their relationships with their patients and with other local practitioners with whom they were involved in varying degrees of cooperation and competition; in England, for example, and despite the existence of the Royal Colleges and the Society of Apothecaries, the medical profession had little effective organisation beyond the local level (Waddington, 1984). Two hundred years later, the figurations in which sports physicians are involved today are much larger, much more complex, and may involve far-flung international relationships involving, among many others, athletes, coaches, team managers, sports promoters, a variety of other sports medicine practitioners (physiotherapists, exercise physiologists, sports psychologists, dietitians, experts in biomechanics, etc.), sports medicine researchers, as well as national and international sports federations and medical organisations, and commercial sponsors; it goes without saying that all these developments have to be seen as aspects of the changing structure of modern sporting competition, a key aspect of which has been the commercialisation of elite sport.

It is, we suggest, not possible to understand the development of modern sports medicine without taking into account these many changes in the structure of sporting competition and the medical profession as well as changes in the structure of the wider society and the ways in which these have impacted upon the relationships between sports physicians and their athlete patients. This is, however, not to say that social processes *determine* developments in medical or scientific knowledge.

All forms of knowledge have a degree of autonomy from other aspects of the social structure although, as Elias pointed out, this degree of autonomy varies considerably from one set of ideas to another, with scientific ideas having a significantly greater degree of autonomy than, for example, political or other ideologies. Elias also noted that some sciences are more autonomous that others, with the natural sciences typically having a higher degree of autonomy than the social sciences, while the degree of autonomy also varies within a science depending on the level of development of that science (Elias, 1978a, 2009c). However, if the figuration of relationships within which practitioners and scientists work cannot be understood as *determining* the structure of their knowledge, it is equally the case that the development of scientific/medical knowledge has to be understood as a social process and that means locating that process of development within the context of – or more precisely, seeing it as an aspect of – the figurations within which practitioners and researchers were involved.

We can further elaborate on this point by reference to another theoretical concept on which we draw. In the 1970s, one of the current authors (I. W.) was involved with two colleagues at Leicester University, Sydney Holloway and Nick Jewson, in developing what was then seen as a distinctive approach, described by some authors as the work of the 'Leicester School' (Woodward and Richards, 1977: 30), to understanding the development of medical knowledge. Central to this approach was the attempt to analyse the figurations in which medical practitioners and medical researchers were involved in the late eighteenth and nineteenth centuries, and the ways in which these figurations inhibited or facilitated the development of particular kinds of medical knowledge. This led to the analysis of three distinctive types of figurations and, associated with each, three distinctive types of medical knowledge or, as Jewson described them, three distinctive 'modes of production of medical knowledge': bedside medicine (Holloway, 1964; Jewson, 1974), hospital medicine (Waddington, 1973) and laboratory medicine (Jewson, 1976). Jewson's (1976) concept, adapted from Marx, of the mode of production of medical knowledge, was defined as involving the following: a group which controls and mobilises the means of production of medical knowledge but is not itself directly involved in the process – the patron(s); a group which, with a greater or lesser degree of relative autonomy, undertakes the process of production of medical knowledge – medical investigators; the network of relations binding patrons and investigators; the raw materials of production – in this case perceptions of the context within which morbid processes occur and within which explanations and cures must be sought; the production process itself – the predominant occupational activity of medical investigators; and the product – a system of theoretical presentations of bodily events (Jewson, 1976: 226–227). The concept of the mode of production is, we suggest, useful in sensitising us to some key aspects of the figurations which are central to understanding the development of science.

In a not dissimilar way to Jewson, Brissonneau (2015) has also drawn upon Marx to describe the 'mode of production of the sporting performance'. In analogous fashion to Jewson's concept of the mode of production of medical knowledge, Brissonneau's concept focuses on the interrelationships between all those involved in producing the sporting performance, involving not just the athletes themselves but also the many others who have come to play an increasingly important part in producing the sporting performance: coaches, trainers, managers, the many specialists within sports medicine as well, of course, as commercial and other sponsors and national governments. Brissonneau himself used the concept to analyse changing patterns of organisation in French cycling from the 'artisanal mode of production' in the 1970s – small scale, consisting of family and former riders, with small budgets, little specialisation and an empiricist approach to training – to the modern structure, based on large budgets from national/international companies which have facilitated much larger and more complex organisational structures involving the employment of many specialists with a high level of division of labour and a highly scientific approach to training. This change in the mode of production of the sporting performance illustrates perfectly a central aspect of modern sport: that elite athletes today are almost invariably surrounded by a whole group of specialist advisers, including specialists in sports medicine. For an understanding of modern sports medicine, it is clearly important to understand the role of sports medicine practitioners, and of sports medical knowledge, in the production of the modern sporting performance.

We need to make one final point about our theoretical standpoint. Throughout this book we have sought to offer a relatively detached analysis of the development of modern sports medicine. We deliberately use the term 'relatively detached' rather than 'objective' because, following Elias (1987b), we believe the concepts of involvement and detachment offer important advantages over the more commonly used terms 'objectivity' and 'subjectivity'.

Elias suggested that one of the problems associated with concepts like objectivity and subjectivity is that they tend to suggest a static and unbridgeable divide between two entities, 'subject' and 'object', and closely associated with this is the almost ubiquitous tendency, among those who use these terms, to describe research in all-or-nothing terms – that is, to describe it as either totally 'objective' or, conversely, as completely lacking in objectivity, that is, as being 'subjective' in an absolute sense.

Clearly, such a conceptualisation is of little use, for – to stick with these terms for the moment – it is impossible to find an example of thinking which is absolutely 'objective' and it is equally difficult to find examples, at least among sane adults, of thinking which is wholly 'subjective' in character. Equally, it is not possible in these terms adequately to describe the development of modern medicine and science, for this development was a long-term social process and there was not a single, historic moment when 'objective' scientific knowledge suddenly emerged, fully formed, out of what had formerly been wholly 'subjective' forms of knowledge.

What is required, argued Elias, is a more adequate conceptualisation of our ways of thinking about the world, and of the social processes as a result of which our present, more scientific, ways of thinking developed. Elias's conceptualisation of the problem in terms of degrees of involvement and detachment is, we would argue, more adequate than conventional conceptualisations because, firstly, it does not involve a radical dichotomy between categories such as 'objective' and 'subjective', as though these were mutually exclusive categories and, secondly, because this conceptualisation is processual – that is, it provides us with a framework with which we can examine the development, over time, of more scientific (or what Elias called more object-adequate or alternatively more reality-congruent) knowledge.

It is important to stress that Elias emphatically rejected the possibility that the outlook of any sane adult can be either wholly detached or wholly involved. Clearly, therefore, Elias did not suggest that it is possible for us to obtain 'ultimate truth', or 'complete detachment'.[1] It is certainly not our claim to offer in this book anything remotely resembling 'ultimate truth' – whatever that might be – or complete detachment; what we hope to offer is a relatively detached perspective which helps to advance, in some small way, our understanding of some key aspects of the relationships between modern sport, sports medicine and the use of performance-enhancing substances or methods.

It is important to stress that it is not our intention to develop a moral critique of sports medicine or of those who practise it, or indeed, of drug use in sport in general. We have written extensively about drug use in modern sport elsewhere and have noted that discussions about this issue are often highly emotive and heavily value-laden, with the consequence that they usually generate more heat than light (Waddington and Smith, 2009: 11). We are sociologists, not moral entrepreneurs, and our task is not to offer a moral critique in which we seek to condemn, but a social scientific analysis in which we seek to understand and explain.

In this connection, it is worth reminding ourselves that, as Elias pointed out, there is an important difference between sociological detachment and emotional and ideological involvement and the proper task of sociologists is not to establish the validity of a preconceived idea about how societies – or, one might add, a particular segment of society such as sports medicine – *ought* to be ordered; rather, the proper task of sociologists is:

> to find connections between particular social events, how their sequence can actually be explained, and what help sociological theories can offer in explaining and determining the trend of social problems – and, last but not least, in providing practical solutions to them.
>
> (Elias, 1978a: 153)

Elias noted that to adopt this approach in our work requires a special effort of detachment. Such an effort may not be easy to make, especially when the subject matter of research touches upon such an emotive issue as drugs, but it is an effort which, both in terms of improved understanding and in terms of responding more effectively to the policy issues involved, is one which is well worth making.

Note

1 Some critics of Elias have argued that advocates of his approach claim to be able to offer 'objective' analyses of social processes. From what has been said, it should be clear that this was not Elias's position and, indeed, it is a position which he explicitly

rejected. However, since some of Elias's critics have misunderstood his position on this point, it may be useful to reiterate one of the arguments contained in his classic essay, 'Problems of involvement and detachment' (1956). Elias noted that sociologists, like everyone else, are members of many social groups outside their academic communities – families, political parties, sports clubs and so on – and they cannot cease to take part in, or to be affected by, the social and political affairs of their groups and their time. In this sense they cannot be wholly detached. However, Elias goes on to note that there is at least one sense in which it would not desirable, in terms of the development of sociology, for them to be wholly detached, even if this were possible. Thus, while one need not know, in order to understand the structure of a molecule, what it feels like to be one of its atoms, in order to understand the way in which human groups work, one needs to know, as it were, from 'inside' how human beings experience their own and other groups, and one cannot know this without actual participation and involvement. The problem for sociologists, then, is not the problem of how to be completely detached, but of how to maintain an appropriate balance between these two roles of everyday participant and scientific inquirer and, as members of a scientific professional group, to establish in their work the undisputed dominance of the latter.

Bibliography

Berg, A. and König, D. (2002), History of sports medicine in Germany with special reference to the University of Freiburg, *Europenan Journal of Sport Science*, 2 (4), 1–7.

Brissonneau, C. (2015), The 1998 Tour de France: Festina, from scandal to an affair in cycling, in V. Møller, I. Waddington and J. Hoberman (eds), *Routledge Handbook of Drugs and Sport*, London, Routledge, 191–192.

Brissonneau, C. and Montez de Oca, J. (2018), *Doping in Elite Sports: Voices of French Sportspeople and Their Doctors, 1950–2010*, London, Routledge.

Dimeo, P. (2007), *A History of Drug Use in Sport 1876–1976*, London, Routledge.

Dubin, The Hon. Charles, L. (1990), *Commission of Inquiry into the Use of Drugs and Banned Practices Intended to Increase Athletic Performance*, Ottawa, Canadian Government Publishing Centre.

Dunning, E. and Waddington, I. (2003), Sport as a drug and drugs in sport: some exploratory comments, *International Review for the Sociology of Sport*, 38 (3), 351–368.

Elias, N. (1956), Problems of involvement and detachment, *British Journal of Sociology*, 7 (3), 226–252.

Elias, N. (1972), Theory of science and history of science, *Economy and Society*, 1 (2), 117–133.

Elias, N. (1978a), *What is Sociology?* London, Hutchinson.

Elias, N. ([1939], 1978b), *The Civilizing Process, Vol. 1: The History of Manners*, Oxford, Blackwell.

Elias, N. (1987a), The retreat of sociologists into the present, *Theory, Culture and Society*, 4 (2–3), 223–247.

Elias, N. (1991), *The Society of Individuals*, Oxford, Blackwell.

Elias, N. (2009a), Social processes, in R. Kilminster and S Mennell (eds), *The Collected Works of Norbert Elias*, Vol. 16, Essays III, Dublin, University College Dublin Press, 4–8

Elias, N. (2009b), Figuration, in R. Kilminster and S Mennell (eds), *The Collected Works of Norbert Elias*, Vol. 16, Essays III, Dublin, University College Dublin Press, 1–3.

Elias, N. (2009c), Sociology of knowledge: New perspectives, in R. Kilminster and S Mennell (eds), *The Collected Works of Norbert Elias*, Vol. 14, Essays I, Dublin, University College Dublin Press, 3–41.

Hansted, D-V., Smith A. and Waddington, I. (2008), The establishment of the world anti-doping agency: a study of organizational change and unplanned outcomes, *International Review for the Sociology of Sport*, 43 (3), 227–249.

Heggie, V. (2011), *A History of British Sports Medicine*, Manchester, Manchester University Press.

Hoberman. J. (1992a), *Mortal Engines: The Science of Performance and the Dehumanization of Sport,* New York, Free Press.

Hoberman, J. (2002), Sports physicians and the doping crisis in elite sport, *Clinical Journal of Sports Medicine,* 12, 203–208.

Hoberman, J. (2012), Sports physicians and doping; medical ethics and elite performance, in D. Malcolm and P. Safai (eds), *The Social Organization of Sports Medicine*, London, Routledge, 237–264.

Hoberman, J. (2013), Sports physicians, human nature, and the limits of medical enhancement, in J. Tolleneer, S. Sterckx and P. Bone (eds), *Athletic Enhancement, Human Nature and Ethics,* Dordrecht, Springer, 255–270.

Holloway, S. W. F. (1964), Medical education in England, 1830–1858: A sociological analysis, *History*, XLIX, 299–324.

Hollman, W. and Tittel, K. (2008), Geshichte der deutschen Sportmedizin, Gera: Druckhaus Gera.

Jewson, N. (1974), Medical knowledge and the patronage system in eighteenth century England, *Sociology*, 8, 369–385.

Jewson, N. (1976), The disappearance of the sick-man from medical cosmology 1770–1870, *Sociology*, 10, 225–244.

Krüger, M. (2015), History of sport medicine in Germany: Some preliminary reflections on a complex research project, *Historical Social Research*, 40 (4), 331–349.

Mclaren, R. H. (2016a), *Independent Person Report: WADA Investigation of Sochi Allegations,* Montreal, WADA.

Mclaren, R. H. (2016b), *Independent Person 2nd Report: WADA Investigation of Sochi Allegations,* Montreal, WADA.

Paoli, L. (2019), The peculiarities of the role of the market for doping products and the role of academic physicians, in B. Fincoeur, J. Gleaves and F. Ohl (eds), *Doping in Cycling: Interdisciplinary Perspectives*, London, Routledge, 79–96.

Paoli, L. and Donati, A. (2014), *The Sports Doping Market: Understanding Supply and Demand and the Challenges of Their Control*, New York, Springer.

Riordan, J. (1991), .*Sport, Politics and Communism*, Manchester, Manchester University Press.

Ryan, A. J. (1989), Sports medicine in the world today, in A. J. Ryan and F. L. Allman, Jr. (eds), *Sports Medicine,* 2nd ed., San Diego, Academic Press, 3–21.

Tipton, C. M. (1997), Sports medicine: A century of progress, *The Journal of Nutrition*, 127 (5), 8788s–885s.

United States Anti-Doping Agency (USADA) (2012), *Reasoned Decision of the United States Anti-Doping Agency on Disqualification and Ineligibility*, Colorado Springs, USADA.

Waddington, I. (1973), The role of the hospital in the development of modern medicine, *Sociology*, 7, 211–224

Waddington, I. (1984), *The Medical Profession in the Industrial Revolution*, Dublin, Gill and Macmillan.

Waddington, I. (1996), The development of sports medicine, *Sociology of Sport Journal*, 13 (2), 176–196.

Waddington, I. (2000), *Sport, Health and Drugs*, London, Spon.

Waddington, I. (2001), Doping in sport: A medical sociological perspective, in *Research on Doping in Sport*, Oslo: Norwegian University of Sport and Physical Education, 11–21.

Waddington, I. (2004), Doping in sport: Some issues for medical practitioners, in J. Hoberman and V. Møller (eds), *Doping and Public Policy*, Odense, University Pres of Southern Denmark, 31–44.

Waddington, I (2005), Le dopage sportif: le responsibilité? des praticiens médicaux/Doping in sport: the responsibilities of medical practitioners, *Revue internationale des sciences du sport et de l'education physique/International Journal of Sport Science and Physical Education*, 26, 9–23.

Waddington, I. (2007), Health and sport, in G. Ritzer (ed.), *The Blackwell Encyclopedia of Sociology*, Oxford, Blackwell, HE-LE., Vol. V, 2091–2095.

Waddington, I. (2015), Towards an understanding of drug use in sport: A medical sociological perspective, in V. Møller, I. Waddington and J. Hoberman (eds), *Routledge Handbook of Drugs and Sport*, London, Routledge, 405–417.

Waddington, I. (2016), Social and behavioural perspectives on drug use in sport, in N. Ahmadi, A. Ljungqvist and G. Svedsäter (eds), *Doping and Public Health*, London: Routledge, 22–37.

Waddington, I. (2019), Changing patterns of drug use in professional cycling: implications for anti-doping policy, in B. Fincoeur, J. Gleaves and F. Ohl (eds), *Doping in Cycling: Interdisciplinary Perspectives*, London, Routledge, 31–44.

Waddington, I. and Møller, V. (2019), WADA at twenty: Old problems and old solutions? *International Journal of Sport Policy and Politics*, 11 (2), 219–231

Waddington, I. and Smith, A. (2009), *An Introduction to Drugs in Sport: Addicted to Winning?* London, Routledge.

Woodward, J. and Richards, D. (1977), Towards a social history of medicine, in J. Woodward and D. Richards (eds), *Health Care and Popular Medicine in Nineteenth Century England*, London, Croom Helm, 15–53.

Part 1

The origins and early development of sports medicine

1 Premodern conceptions of exercise and health

At the outset, we should note a point of central importance: from the ancient world until the mid-nineteenth century, physicians were the only occupational group with a professional interest in exercise, which meant that physicians had an effective monopoly in terms of defining the meaning and significance of exercise. We shall see the full significance of this in the next chapter. But firstly, of what did this corpus of medical knowledge consist?

As we noted earlier, the development of sports medicine in the form in which we know it today, that is as a specialised body of knowledge and practice within the medical profession with its own institutional structure, is a relatively recent process which dates from the twentieth century. However, numerous scholars have suggested that the origins of sports medicine can be traced back much further than this. Ryan (1989: 3), for example, has suggested that 'sports medicine has developed gradually, though sporadically, over a period of 2500 years'. It is certainly the case that physicians in the ancient world recognised a positive association between exercise and health (MacAuley, 1994; American Academy of Orthopaedic Surgeons, 1984; Aneni and Adegoju, 2019; Lazovic, 2015; Hill, 2019; Ergen, 2016) and Berryman (1992, 2010, 2012a), in particular, has documented in some detail the enduring legacy of classical Greek medicine in this respect.

Recognition of the health benefits of moderate exercise can be traced back to at least Hippocrates and Galen (Berryman, 1992). Exercise played a significant part in the general medical theory – known as humoural theory – which was developed by these two ancient physicians and which, throughout the eighteenth century, was generally referred to as 'Galenic medical theory'. Galen structured his theory around the so-called 'naturals' (things of, or with, nature – e.g. human physiology), the 'non-naturals' (things not innate – e.g. hygiene) and the contra-naturals (things against nature – pathology). An important element of Galenic theory were the six non-naturals: (i) air; (ii) food and drink; (iii) motion and rest; (iv) sleep and wake; (v) excretions and retentions; (vi) passions of the mind. Central to humoural theory was the idea that a proper balance between the four humours (blood – hot and moist; phlegm – cold and moist, yellow bile – hot and dry; and black bile – cold and dry) characterised a healthy body and mind, while an imbalance led to disease. The non-naturals, Galen argued, should be used in moderation and if taken in excess would result in an imbalance which could lead to disease. In this context, it might be noted that Galen did not endorse the athletic activities of the classical world

DOI: 10.4324/9781003563921-3

(Ryan, 1989: 6). He criticised what he described as 'the unnatural state of athletes' (Hoberman, 1992: 105), suggesting that athletes neglected 'the old rule of health which prescribes moderation in all things', that they 'exceed the proper measure in exertion', are 'in miserable pain' and that, when they stop competing, 'most parts of their bodies become deformed' (cited in Berryman, 2012a: 211). The stress on moderate exercise, coupled with warnings of the dangers of 'excessive' exercise, were to be recurring features in later medical views of the relationships between exercise and health.

In Galenic theory, the role of exercise and rest related to their supposed effects on the qualities (hot, cold, moist and dry) of the four humours. It was believed that excessive rest increased cold and moisture, whereas excessive exercise would initially heat the body, to be followed by cold and dryness. Moderate exercise maintained warmth while baths of different temperatures were also recommended for their coolness, dryness or heating capabilities. Since disease was held to be caused by an imbalance between the qualities of the four humours, and since these were thought to be influenced by rest and exercise, the latter were regarded as key elements of the non-naturals and were incorporated in much of the early literature on regimen which, for several centuries, was a central component in medical thought, especially on preventive medicine (Berryman, 1992: 2–4, 2010: 195).

Berryman (1992: 16–35) has noted that there was a revival of medical interest in the non-naturals in sixteenth- and seventeenth-century Europe, and a further expansion of the non-natural theme in eighteenth-century medicine. He notes that the Greek principles of hygiene and regimen, which included exercise as one of the non-naturals, 'continued to flourish in 18th century Europe' (Berryman, 2010: 196), and that classical Greek preventive hygiene 'was part of formal medical training through the eighteenth century' (Berryman, 1992: 3).

Park (1992: 61) has similarly noted that at the beginning of the nineteenth century, 'the "non-naturals", classical therapeutics, and traditional theories of hygiene still exerted a major influence on concepts of health and disease' and she adds that 'Galen remained the standard authority'.

In relation to the development of medical knowledge more generally, Jewson has similarly noted the persistence of key elements of classical Galenic medical theory throughout the era of 'bedside medicine', that is until roughly the end of the eighteenth century. Jewson (1974: 370–371) has noted that the works of classical authors enjoyed great authority in fifteenth- and sixteenth-century Europe, and that even the seventeenth-century scientific revolution had little impact on the fundamental characteristics of medical theory and therapy. In this regard, he notes that one particularly powerful influence on medical thought from the mid-seventeenth century was that of Newtonian physics, which enjoyed high prestige in both scientific and non-scientific circles, and the elite of the medical profession accordingly sought to import its fashionable ideas into their theories. However, he suggests that most of the medical authors who invoked the name of Newton had little understanding of his ideas, while there were also a number of different interpretations of his ideas in circulation. The result was that:

> the introduction of Newtonianism into medicine did not herald a thoroughgoing reformulation of theories of pathology. Instead it gave a new lease of life to the ancient conceptions of disease which reappeared under a new guise. The basic entities of the humoural system were re-defined in terms of material entities, such as corpuscular flow, or excitement of the muscles, but the general conception of the bodily system propounded by Hippocrates and Galen remained the guiding principle of research and practice ... despite criticism of specific aspects of the ancient texts and the appeal to new sources of legitimation, the classical authors remained the standard works read by medical students at the English universities.
>
> (Jewson, 1974: 371–372)

How, then, can we explain this persistence, until the late eighteenth century, of these classical systems of medical thought, of which the non-naturals were a part? There are two key general points here: firstly, medical knowledge must be viewed 'as a form of social interaction between the sick and medical personnel' (Jewson, 1974: 369) and, secondly, that 'one of the major constraints operating on the producers of any product is the structure of the market for that product' (Waddington, 1984: 180). In this regard, it is important to note that in eighteenth-century Europe the demand for the services of physicians was very limited and highly concentrated among the higher status groups within the population. As Holloway (1964) has noted, in the eighteenth century the aristocratic and wealthy patient was the dominant figure in the doctor-patient relationship; that is, the relationship was one of patronage. By virtue of the wider social basis of their power, the patient was in a position to define both their own needs and the manner in which those needs were to be met. Thus 'the patient, not the doctor, determined the conditions on which service was rendered. The client demanded a cure; the practitioner was in no position to suspend judgement and proceed with caution. He had to act quickly; treatment had to be given and conclusions drawn from partial evidence or even pure speculation'. Thus the doctor, 'faced by powerful, wealthy, critical, demanding and ill-informed patients, was forced into the role of lackey and mere comforter' (Holloway, 1964: 301–302).

Under such conditions, client control was maximised and the technically based authority of the physician minimised; indeed technical competence was not the major criterion in terms of which practitioners were evaluated. The eighteenth-century physician was expected to be, above all else, a gentleman, socially accepted in the circles among which his patrons moved. Elegance and wit were of greater importance than technical competence.[1] As Jewson (1974: 376) has noted, within this structure 'the nobility and gentry held sway over the medical profession', not least because 'success in a medical career, as in other occupations, depended on the cultivation of close personal ties with members of the upper class'.

This structure of medical practice was inimical to medical innovation in several ways. Jewson (1974: 377) has noted that the influence of the upper-class patients may be seen in the high status accorded to philosophical speculation by eighteenth-century physicians for, in 'an age in which upper class education and culture were founded in classical literature the prestige attached to the work of Hippocrates and Galen is obvious'. In this context it should be noted that although of lesser status than his patients, the eighteenth-century physician – unlike the lower status surgeons (or barber-surgeons) and apothecaries – was nevertheless considered to be a scholar and a gentleman and his education in the classical medical literature was a key aspect of this status differentiation (Waddington, 1984).

But the structure of medical practice in the eighteenth century also placed constraints on the pursuit of scientific medical research in other, more direct, ways. Jewson (1974) notes that, at this time, there was no differentiation between the social roles of therapist and research worker.[2] Consequently medical investigators were unable to attain that degree of detachment from the opinions of patients which was necessary to foster a scientific approach to theory and practice. Moreover, there was little incentive for physicians to engage in research, since this offered little in terms of career advantage; in the eighteenth-century medical careers were furthered not so much by making basic discoveries as by making new friends in the appropriate social circles. For their part, physicians were unlikely to risk the lives – and the invaluable patronage – of wealthy and influential private patients with new and untried therapies while, in addition – and this constitutes perhaps the most serious obstacle to innovation – such patients were unlikely to be willing to act as guinea pigs for new, and perhaps uncomfortable and potentially dangerous, techniques: the patient had the power of the veto. Fundamental innovations in the structure of medical thought and practice had to wait upon radical changes in the doctor-patient relationship, which were a key part of the development of a new mode of production of medical knowledge, in the early nineteenth century (Waddington, 1973).

Not surprisingly, these classically based speculative medical systems of the eighteenth century offered little by way of effective therapies and Berryman (2010: 195) has suggested that the relative absence of known cures may account, in part, for the stress which was laid on a regimen of preventive medicine and hygiene, including exercise, in the medical literature until the early nineteenth century. He notes that while exercise was recommended for some illnesses, 'the primary use of exercise was for prophylaxis' (Berryman, 2010: 195). Krüger (2015: 335) has similarly pointed to the importance of exercise as an aspect of preventive medicine at this time, noting that the 'obligation of a doctor was essentially to "keep the body healthy", and less to cure diseases'. However, in the course of the nineteenth century, the balance between cure and prevention in medical practice, and with it the emphasis on exercise as a form of prevention, began to shift. But this shift in the balance between prevention and cure was not the only process which relegated exercise to the margins of medical practice; of no less importance was the development in the nineteenth century of modern sport, for this was associated with the emergence of occupational groups which offered new and non-medical definitions of the meaning and significance of sport, which effectively deprived physicians of their longstanding monopoly in this area. We explore these developments in the next chapter.

Notes

1 Thus in England, practitioners such as Sir Samuel Garth, Mark Akenside and John Arbuthnot were as noted for their literary writing as for their medical publications, while others, such as Richard Brocklesby and Richard Mead, were patrons of the arts and were on intimate terms with the wits and poets of the period. For full biographical details of these physicians, see the *Dictionary of National Biography*. For other examples, including many from other parts of Europe, see A. Castiglioni: *A History of Medicine* (New York, 1947), pp. 654–655, and F. H. Garrison: *An Introduction to the History of Medicine* (Philadelphia and London, 1929), pp. 381–389. It is interesting to note that in England, this emphasis on the social graces rather than on technical competence, persisted until well into the nineteenth century. In Anthony Trollope's *Doctor Thorne*, first published in 1858, Lady Arabella, wife of the Squire of Greshamsbury prefers to have as her medical attendant the gentlemanly Dr Fillgrave rather than the 'half-apothecary' Dr Thorne, despite the fact that Dr Thorne is the more competent practitioner.

2 Jewson (1974: 385) notes that those who engaged in both activities sometimes had to endure role conflicts. He notes that William Harvey 'seems to have resolved his difficulties by maintaining a strict segregation between his therapeutic and scientific interests. Thus the discoverer of the circulation of the blood continued, in his professional capacity, to strongly recommend bloodletting which he justified by appeal to a Galenic rationale'. See also K.D. Keele, *William Harvey: The Man, the Physician, and The Scientist* (London, Nelson, 1965), pp. 80–81.

References

American Academy of Orthopaedic Surgeons (1984), Pioneers in sports medicine, in *Athletic Training and Sports Medicine,* Chicago, American Academy of Sports Medicine, 3–6.

Aneni, M. O. and Adegoju, F. A. (2019), Exercise in antiquity and modern times: Catholicon for healthy living, *African Research Review*, 13 (1), 39–50.

Berryman, J. W. (1992), Exercise and the medical tradition from Hippocrates through Antebellum America, in J. W. Berryman and R. J. Park (eds), *Sport and Exercise Medicine: Essays in the History of Sports Medicine*, Urbana and Chicago, University of Illinois Press, 1–56.

Berryman, J. W. (2010), Exercise is medicine: An historical perspective, *Current Sports Medicine Reports*, 9 (4), 195–201.

Berryman, J. W. (2012a), The art of medicine: Galen on exercise and health, *Lancet*, 380, 210–211.

Ergen, E. (2016), The origins of sports medicine, *Aspetar Sports Medicine Review*, 5 (2), 342–348.

Hill, L. (2019), Exercise science and sport medicine: An ancient account, *Russian Journal of Physical Education and Sport*, 14 (2), 93–97.

Hoberman, J. (1992), *Mortal Engines: The Science of Performance and the Dehumanization of Sport,* New York, Free Press.

Holloway, S. W. F. (1964), Medical education in England, 1830–1858: A sociological analysis, *History*, XLIX, 299–324.

Jewson, N. (1974), Medical knowledge and the patronage system in eighteenth century England, *Sociology*, 8, 369–385.

Kruger, M. (2015), History of sport medicine in Germany. Some preliminary reflections on a complex research project, *Historical Social Research*, 40 (4), 331–349.

Lazovic, B. (2015), Sports medicine: A historical perspective with special reference to Eastern Europe, *Aspetar Sports Medicine Journal*, 3, 574–581.

MacAuley, D. (1994), A history of physical activity, health and medicine, *Journal of the Royal Society of Medicine,* 87, 32–35.

Park, R. J. (1992), Athletes and their training in Britain and America, 1800–1914, in J. B. Berryman and R. J. Park (eds), *Sport and Exercise Medicine: Essays in the History of Sports Medicine*, Urban and Chicago, University of Illinois Press, 57–107.

Ryan, A. J. (1989), Sports medicine in the world today, in A. J. Ryan and F. L. Allman, Jr. (eds), *Sports Medicine,* 2nd ed., San Diego, Academic Press, 3–21.

Waddington, I. (1973), The role of the hospital in the development of modern medicine, *Sociology*, 7, 211–224.

Waddington, I. (1984), *The Medical Profession in the Industrial Revolution*, Dublin, Gill and Macmillan.

2 The development of modern sport and the marginalisation of exercise in nineteenth century medicine

In the course of the nineteenth century, exercise became increasingly marginal to mainstream medical practice as a result of two major developments: the development of modern sport and the development of modern medicine.

Sport as a game changer

As Elias (1986a, 1986b) has noted, in the course of the nineteenth century – and in some cases as early as the mid-eighteenth century – with England as the model-setting country, some leisure activities involving bodily exertion assumed the structural characteristics which we identify with modern sports. This sportisation process, as Elias called it, was a 'game changer' in relation to the development of sports medicine, not only in the obvious sense that, in the longer term, it provided a group of people who came to constitute the patient group for the development of a new medical specialism but also because, in the shorter term, it was associated with the development of non-medical occupational groups with a professional interest in sport who offered new definitions of the meaning and significance of sport which challenged the longstanding monopoly of physicians in this area.

As numerous scholars have noted, educational institutions were central to the development of modern sport. Dunning and Sheard ([1979] 2005), in what is properly recognised as a classic study, have documented the incipient modernisation of the two forms of football – association football (soccer) and rugby – in the English public schools in the second quarter of the nineteenth century. But the significance of sport within the public schools and the ancient English universities was much more general. Holt (1989: 74) has noted that, if we wish to explain the 'style and spirit in which the new sports were played' and, perhaps more importantly, the cultural centrality they came to have, 'we must look to the growth of the public school and the distinctive range of ideas brought to bear on secondary and higher education in the mid-nineteenth century'. Particularly important in this regard was the 'cult of athleticism' which developed as a central component of the whole system of elite education (Mangan, 1981). At the universities of Oxford and Cambridge, colleges 'became almost as serious about their prowess in sport as the public schools and furnished themselves with similarly splendid facilities', a process in which they were 'merely reflecting the public school devotion to games' (Holt, 1989: 76–83).

DOI: 10.4324/9781003563921-4

These developments were of major significance, not least because, as McIntosh (1968: 33; emphasis added) has noted, in the English public schools games 'were organised and won recognition as a *means of education*'. Central to what Mangan (1981) has accurately described as an 'educational ideology' was the idea that sport, and in particular team games, were essential for the achievement of key educational – and specifically moral – goals. In 1854, former pupils of Winchester School set out in a memorandum what they considered the benefits of team games; they were, they said, 'a preparation for the battle of life, that they trained moral qualities, namely respect for others, patient endurance, unflagging courage, self-reliance and self-control, vigour and decisiveness of character "to which England owes much of her greatness"' (cited in McIntosh, 1968: 45). The 1864 Report of the Clarendon Commission, appointed to inquire into the management of nine major public schools, similarly recognised the educational value of organised games in training character, and that the cricket and football fields helped to form 'some of the most valuable social qualities and manly virtues' (McIntosh, 1968: 49–50). The development of this ideology was of major significance, for it meant that the key element of these newly emerging forms of modern sport was defined not in relation to health but, rather, in relation to their educational, and specifically their *moral* purpose. And central to this process was the fact that the definition of the meaning and significance of exercise, in the form of modern sport, was beginning to shift away from the province of medicine and towards that of education, that is, away from physicians and towards the newly emerging occupational group of games masters, of whom a growing number were appointed in the public schools in the late nineteenth century (McIntosh, 1968: 59), and who represented the incipient development of physical education within the teaching profession.

Of course it was not just in England that educational institutions played a major part in the development of sport. In the United States, too, the colleges were one of the most important sources for the development of modern sports (Waddington and Roderick, 1996). Prior to the Civil War there were already some 250 colleges in the United States and in the second half of the nineteenth century, sport came to play an increasingly important part in the American college system, a part which, in some respects, was not unlike that played by the 'games cult' in the English public schools. Mandell (1984: 187) has noted that the so-called 'sports craze' on American college campuses in the 1890s was reflected in the development of baseball, rowing, and track and field but, above all, in the development of American football, a process in which the eastern elite universities – Princeton, Columbia, Harvard and Yale – and later the universities of the Middle West, played a central part.

And, as in the case of sports which developed in the English public schools, in the United States too, the newly developing sports derived their meaning and significance not from within a medical context, that is in terms of their relation to health, but in an educational context, in terms of their contribution to 'character formation' – however defined – and to wider social and moral values such as what were then considered to be appropriate models of masculinity and, perhaps particularly important in what was still a relatively new nation, the contribution of what were held to be distinctively American sports to the development of an American national identity (Waddington and Roderick, 1996). In this regard, Berryman (2010: 197) has noted that in pre-Civil War America, physicians had used the term 'physical education' to indicate the task of teaching the traditional 'Laws of Health', which included recognition of exercise as one of the 'non-naturals' which influenced health. However, the development of modern sport led, in America as in Britain, to physicians ceding control of the definition of the meaning and significance of sport to educators over the next half century or so. Berryman notes that

> What began in the late 1850s as the Muscular Christianity Movement, where high moral standards of character, citizenship, and sportsmanship were viewed as valuable by-products of team participation, gained momentum throughout the last half of the 19th century through college and high school sports and the YMCA.

Baseball, football, track and field, swimming and tennis became the new subject matter of physical education, while physical education in high schools and colleges came increasingly to be regarded as 'education through the physical' rather than 'education of the physical'. Moreover, Berryman (2010: 197) points out that 'to teach and coach these new games, schools and colleges needed men and women with expertise in one or more sports, not physicians'. As a result of these and similar developments within the American educational system, 'the moral and educational benefits of playing games overshadowed their health promotion values', as physical education became not a health-based curriculum but a sports skills curriculum. Berryman (2010: 198) adds that the

> 'Sports Creed' emphasising citizenship, teamwork, character, democratic living, and sportsmanship had replaced the 'Laws of Health' as the focal point for physical education … the new physical education curriculum, focusing on competitive sports required the hiring of coaches, not physicians, and favored those students blessed with physicality, providing very little exercise for those not so fortunate.

The result was that 'physical education' in the United States changed to a games and sports curriculum led by coaches who introduced competition and athletic achievement into the classroom, and 'as that happened, physicians disappeared from the profession' (Berryman, 2010: 195). Elsewhere, Berryman (2012b: 26–27) has noted that in the late nineteenth and early twentieth centuries, 'organized college sports were becoming popular in the US. The success and widespread interest in athletics at universities began to direct the physical educator's attention away from various exercise systems and calisthenics to games and sports at the expense of health and fitness'.

In addition, as sports became increasingly competitive in the late nineteenth and early twentieth centuries (Dunning, 1986), so the emphasis placed on the acquisition of skills also increased. The English public schools began to employ not just games masters but also professional coaches (McIntosh, 1968: 59) as did the American colleges, some of which were described as having an 'army of professional coaches and trainers' (Paine, 1905, cited in Park, 1992: 83). And the development of coaching was associated with the emergence of a third definition of the meaning and significance of sport; for coaches, the defining feature of sport was not its relation to health, nor even primarily its relation to character formation *per se*, but rather, the fact that it was a skills-based, competitive activity. As Holt (1989: 87) has noted, sport gradually ceased to be a means to an end, whether defined in terms of the promotion of health or the development of 'character', and 'became an end in itself'. The monopoly which the medical profession, as the only occupational group with a professional interest in the area, had long enjoyed in terms of defining the meaning and significance of exercise, was thus steadily undermined from the mid-nineteenth century, as the locus for defining the significance of sport shifted from medicine to education and, later, coaching. Moreover, and as part of this shift, the role of teachers and coaches within sport became increasingly important as they became gatekeepers, controlling access to participation in the newly emerging forms of modern sport in a way in which physicians had never controlled access to traditional forms of exercise such as walking, riding and hunting.

But if exercise became increasingly marginal in medical practice from the middle of the nineteenth century, this was not simply because physicians were 'pushed out' by the rise of new occupational groups with a professional, non-medical interest in sport, for physicians' dwindling professional interest in exercise was also associated with developments within medicine itself. Central among these was the development of modern medicine from the early nineteenth century which radically transformed the basis of medical knowledge and the practice of medicine, not least in terms of the balance between cure and prevention.

Hospital medicine: a new mode of production of medical knowledge

The advent of modern medicine has been ascribed to a variety of times and places, but medical historians have made a good case for the suggestion that the foundations of modern medicine were laid in Paris in the early part of the nineteenth century (Shryock, 1947, 1957; Ackerknecht, 1967; Rosen, 1956). The major developments in medical knowledge at this time and the changes in the structure of relationships within medicine which facilitated these developments – that is, the new mode of production of medical knowledge – have been analysed in detail elsewhere (Waddington, 1973) and only a short summary is required here.

In relation to medical knowledge, a key process was a methodological change of major significance, involving the shift from observation to examination; there is a good deal of truth in the oft-repeated phrase that prior to 1800 physicians *observed* their patients, subsequently they *examined* them. This shift from observation to examination was associated with several other key innovations: the development of the concept of a localised pathology, based on the techniques of physical examination and autopsy, and the delineation of disease entities by means of correlating external symptoms with internal lesions.

In relation to the structure of medical practice which facilitated these innovations, the key process was the development of a large-scale hospital system in

Paris in the late eighteenth and early nineteenth centuries. This created a large body of 'research material' in the form of large numbers of patients, which provided clinicians with the opportunity to see many more patients and created much greater opportunities for research than had ever been possible in private practice; one Parisian clinician, J. B. Bouillard, saw no fewer than 25,000 cases in a three-year period (Shryock, 1957: 886). However, and of even greater importance, was that the development of the hospital system led to a radical change in the balance of power in the doctor-patient relationship which, for the first time, gave doctors almost unfettered access to the bodies of their patients.

In this context, the shift from observation to examination was not unproblematic, for it required physicians to have access to the bodies of their patients. However, the consent of patients to new, and perhaps uncomfortable and dangerous procedures cannot be assumed but has to be explained. We noted in the previous chapter that, under the patronage system, not only were there few incentives for physicians to engage in research, since this meant little in terms of career advancement, but there were also almost insuperable practical obstacles to be overcome in terms of conducting research on private patients: not only were physicians unwilling to risk the lives – and the invaluable patronage – of powerful, wealthy and influential private patients but such patients were unlikely to be willing to act as guinea pigs for new and untried techniques. Hence a key question has to be answered: why was it that patients in the Paris hospitals offered no resistance to the new, experimental medicine?

The answer, put simply, is that hospital patients were in no position to offer resistance; they had to take what was offered. The most cursory glance at the situation of doctors holding hospital appointments and that of their patients reveals a marked status difference in favour of doctors. Hospital doctors comprised the elite group of medical practitioners, for hospital positions were even more highly prized than university appointments (Ackerknecht, 1967: 15). Not only did they have a virtual monopoly of research facilities, but their status within the hospitals enabled them to attract the wealthiest private patients.

In marked contrast was the situation of hospital patients, who were not only sick, but generally poor too. Conditions in hospitals, and in particular the danger of cross-infection, were sufficient to repel all those who could afford treatment at home. Mac-Auliffe (1901: 222) cites some contemporary (1793) observations to the effect that 'Les hôpitaux étaient véritablement "cet entassement de malades qui les rendent souvent plus dangereux que la maladie elle-même"'. Tenon, writing in 1788, described four, five or six patients to a bed in a major Paris hospital, and 'convalescents together with the sick, the dying and the dead … a room for convalescents on the third floor which could be reached only via the smallpox ward' (cited in Ackerknecht, 1967: 16). The mortality rate at the Hôtel Dieu hospital in 1816 was 1:4.57, while for the period 1805–1814 the mortality rate at the Hôpital Saint Antoine was 1:5.5 and that of the Hôpital de la Charité was 1:7 (Stewart, 1843: 34–47). Hospitals were not places to which one went through choice; they housed those who could not afford to pay a medical practitioner and who had no domicile, or no kin to care for them in illness.

The relatively powerless position of hospital patients was nicely pointed up by Campbell Stewart, who wrote that patients 'must comply, unhesitatingly, with their advice, and abide by the direction of the medical officers; if the slightest difficulty occurs they are immediately discharged'. Even more revealing, perhaps, are his comments on the problems of securing the consent of patients to surgical operations which, at this time, were both extremely dangerous and, frequently, excruciatingly painful. 'It is', he wrote, 'always optional with them to submit to a proposed operation or decline it, but in cases where such operation is considered requisite, they must submit or leave the hospital' (Campbell Stewart, 1843: 98). It is clear that where patients were not in a situation to obtain medical care from an alternative source – that is by employing a practitioner privately – they had little choice but to 'submit'. It might be noted that even Campbell Stewart's choice of terms – notably his reference to patients 'submitting' to the prescribed therapy, nicely brings out the dominance of the doctor in the doctor-patient relationship. The contrast between the comparatively powerful position of the eighteenth-century patron and the comparatively powerless position of the early nineteenth-century hospital patient is so stark as to require no further comment.[1]

The hospital thus provided a practice situation within which, for the first time, doctors were in a position to ignore the wishes of patients where those wishes ran counter to the doctors' professional judgement. Doctors could now define the problems, and the manner in which those problems were to be solved, according to criteria established by the profession, not by the patient. The doctor, in short, was no longer the 'lackey and mere comforter of the rich'.

The availability of a more-or-less captive body of 'research material' in the form of a large and highly vulnerable and potentially exploitable population of hospital patients provided the basis for radical developments in the diagnosis and understanding of disease processes. No longer was disease conceptualised, as in classical eighteenth-century bedside medicine, in terms of total symptom complexes and a systemic imbalance in the whole body, but in terms of specific internal events, local lesions which could be correlated with external symptoms. And although these developments did not, in the immediate short term, generate a large number of new and more effective therapies, they did offer a much more adequate understanding of disease processes which provided the basis for the subsequent development of more effective cures, a process which was further boosted by the possibility of more effective and safer surgery following the development of anaesthetics and antisepsis from the middle years of the nineteenth century. In brief, medical practice was radically transformed in the course of the nineteenth century.

These developments within medicine were, of course, taking place concurrently with the development of modern forms of sport in the nineteenth century, described earlier. Thus, at the very time that other occupational groups were taking a greater interest in sport and – more significantly – offering new and competing non-medical definitions of the meaning and significance of sport, so within medical practice the development of more effective cures was leading to a shift in the balance between cure and prevention. As Berryman (2010: 195) has noted, Western medicine became more focused on 'sick care' with a concomitant loss of the traditional interest in the preventive effects of exercise. He notes that, in America in the early years of the twentieth century, medical education was reorganised to take account of these developments in medicine: 'the course of study became longer, the curriculum became more scientific, a greater emphasis was placed on cure rather than prevention, residency programs were instituted, and most physicians began to specialise'. One outcome was that few physicians looked at 'physical education' as a field of potential employment or one where their expertise would be best utilised or appreciated. 'Accordingly', Berryman (2010: 197) notes, 'exercise began to lose the attention previously displayed by many physicians'. Elsewhere Berryman (2012b: 27) has noted that

> mainstream medicine abandoned its long-standing central component of prevention in favour of new techniques of therapy that were dependent on drugs and surgery … Those with medical training who had once led the movement for systematic exercise moved into mainstream therapy as a career rather than dwelling on the preventive tactics that were so popular before new drugs and surgeries were developed.

A similar point has been made by Ryan, who points out that, in the early part of the nineteenth century, exercise continued to be a mainstay of medical practice, 'since there were relatively few specifics that were effective in spite of the enormous empiric pharmacopeia'. However, he adds that, 'As the century progressed, with the discovery of practical general anesthesia, the formulation of the bacterial origin of infectious disease by Pasteur, the development of antisepsis by Lister, and the foundation of modern chemotherapy by Ehrlich, physicians turned their attention away from exercise and toward the application of these new findings of therapy' (Ryan, 1989: 10). Indeed, not only was it the case that exercise became marginalised within the practice of medicine but, as we shall see, it was also the case that many medical practitioners, as well as many researchers in the developing discipline of exercise physiology, were not only sceptical about the health benefits of modern sports, but many of them warned of what they saw as the health risks associated with participation in these sports.

In most countries, it was to be very many years – indeed, not until the very last years of the twentieth century – before exercise was once again to become an established part of medical thought and practice in relation to the promotion of the health of the general population. The development of modern sports medicine, as we shall see, was to take place in a very different social context: that of high-performance sport. Heggie (2011: 12) has noted that her book, *A History of British Sports Medicine*, focuses on 'elite (national level and above) athletes, and consequently school groups, physical culture and exercise for health are marginalised in this story'. She adds:

> This is not just my prejudice; it is clear that the first institutions of British sports medicine focused on the elite body at the expense of the schoolchild or casual sportsperson. It could have been possible for sports medicine to be constructed as a version of public health or healthy living, but that is not … what happened in Britain.

And, as we shall see, it is not what happened in most other countries. Modern sports medicine was unambiguously the child, not of public health, but of elite sport.

Note

1 Perhaps a more extreme example, from a different society, which illustrates even more clearly the way in which the vulnerability of the patient is socially structured, is provided by the development of gynaecology in America in the middle years of the nineteenth century and particularly by the work of J. Marion Sims who, in 1849, performed the first successful operation for vesico-vaginal fistula. Significantly, all of Sims' experimental operations were performed on slaves. Sims agreed with the owners of the slaves that if they would give him the slaves 'for experiment', he would keep them at his own expense. Some of these slaves Sims kept for as long as four years, during which he performed numerous operations on them; one woman had as many as thirty operations in all. See J. Marion Sims, *The Story of My Life,* New York, 1884, reprinted 1968, 226–246.

References

Ackerknecht, E. H. (1967), *Medicine at the Paris Hospital, 1794–1848*. Baltimore, Johns Hopkins Press.

Berryman, J. W. (2010), Exercise is medicine: An historical perspective, *Current Sports Medicine Reports*, 9 (4), 195–201.

Berryman, J. (2012b), The role of physiology and cardiology in the founding and early years of the American college of sports medicine, in D. Malcolm, and P. Safai (eds), *The Social Organization of Sports Medicine*, New York, Routledge, 25–53.

Dunning, E. (1986), The dynamics of modern sports: Notes on achievement-striving and the social significance of sport, in N. Elias and E. Dunning, *Quest for Excitement: Sport and Leisure in the Civilizing Process*, Oxford, Blackwell, 205–223.

Dunning, E. and Sheard, K. ([1979] 2005), *Barbarians, Gentlemen and Players: A Sociological Study of the Development of Rugby Football*, 2nd ed., London, Routledge.

Elias, N. (1986a) The genesis of sport as a sociological problem, in N. Elias and E. Dunning (eds), *Quest for Excitement: Sport and Leisure in the Civilizing Process,* Oxford, Blackwell, 126–149.

Elias, N. (1986b), An essay on sport and violence, in N. Elias and E. Dunning (eds), *Quest for Excitement: Sport and Leisure in the Civilizing Process,* Oxford, Blackwell, 150–174.

Heggie, V. (2011), *A History of British Sports Medicine*, Manchester, Manchester University Press.

Holt, R. (1989), *Sport and the British: A Modern History*, Oxford, Clarendon Press.

Mac-Auliffe, L. (1901), *La Révolution et les hôpitaux de Paris*, Paris, Société nouvelle de librairie et d'édition.

MacIntosh, P. (1968), *Physical Education in England since 1800*, London, Bell.

Mandell, R. (1984), *Sport: A Cultural History*, New York, Columbia University Press.

Mangan, J. A. (1981), *Athleticism in the Victoria and Edwardian Public School – the Emergence and Consolidation of an Educational Ideology*, Cambridge, Cambridge University Press.

Park, R. J. (1992), Athletes and their training in Britain and America, 1800–1914, in J. B. Berryman and R. J. Park (eds), *Sport and Exercise Medicine: Essays in the History of Sports Medicine*, Urban and Chicago, University of Illinois Press, 57–107.

Paine, R. D. (1905), The spirit of school and college sport: American and English rowing, *The Century Magazine*, 70, 483–503.

Rosen, G. (1956), Hospitals, medical care and social policy in the French Revolution, *Bulletin of the History of Medicine*, 30, 124–149.

Ryan, A. J. (1989), Sports medicine in the world today, in A. J. Ryan and F. L. Allman, Jr. (eds), *Sports Medicine,* 2nd ed., San Diego, Academic Press, 3–21.
Shryock, R. H. (1947), *The Development of Modern Medicine*, New York, Alfred A. Knopf.
Shryock, R. H. (1957), Nineteenth century medicine: Scientific aspects, *Journal of World History*, 3, 881–908.
Stewart, F. C. (1843), *The Hospitals and Surgeons of Paris*, New York, J. and H. G. Langley
Waddington, I. (1973), The role of the hospital in the development of modern medicine, *Sociology*, 7, 211–224.
Waddington, I. and Roderick, M. (1996), American exceptionalism: Soccer and American football, *The Sports Historian*, 16, 42–63.

3 The incipient development of sports medicine

The period from the late nineteenth century through the first three decades of the twentieth century was an important period in the incipient development of modern sports medicine. During this period there were three processes, in particular, which require detailed analysis. These were: the development of the modern laboratory-based discipline of exercise physiology; the limited provision of some sort of medical care to some elite athletes by a variety of practitioners, most of whom had no medical qualifications but who did include a small but growing number of doctors; and the movement towards the establishment of more formal organisational structures by physicians with an interest in sport, a development which culminated in 1928 in the foundation of the Association Internationale Médico-Sportive (AIMS), which in 1934 became the Fédération Internationale de Médecine Sportive, the name which it has retained ever since. The first two processes are examined in this chapter while the third process is the focus of the next chapter.

The development of exercise physiology

As we saw in the previous chapter, in the course of the nineteenth century exercise lost much of its salience within the day-to-day practice of medicine. From the middle years of the nineteenth century, those involved in the everyday practice of medicine were also marginalised in relation to research into the physiological effects of exercise, as the key function of developing scientific knowledge in this area became institutionalised in the newly emerging discipline of exercise physiology.

The structural basis for the new science was laboratory medicine, which was first established within the German university system in the middle decades of the nineteenth century. The two major initial areas of development were histology, in which numerous discoveries concerning the properties of tissues were organised into a coherent synthesis by the development of cell theory and, of more direct relevance for our concerns here, experimental physiology (Jewson, 1976: 230). France, too, made a significant contribution to these developments; as Heggie (2016: 198) has noted, 'in continental Europe, particularly in Germany and France, the institutions and facilities for laboratory-based experimental physiology appeared considerably before equivalent institutions in the United Kingdom or the United States'.

The development of laboratory medicine represented a third 'mode of production of medical knowledge' (after bedside medicine and hospital medicine) which

DOI: 10.4324/9781003563921-5

involved, as a central characteristic, what Jewson (1976) has described as the 'disappearance of the sick-man from medical cosmology', that is, the disappearance of the sick person as the central focus of the investigators' research activity. Under the traditional system of bedside medicine, the dominant perspective was that of the powerful patron/patient who was in a position to define both their own needs and the manner in which those needs were to be met. With the development of hospital medicine in the early nineteenth century, medical practitioners were, as we have seen, able to gain a substantial degree of social distance from their patients, which enabled the clinical gaze – with an emphasis on new diagnostic techniques based on physical examination, new research methods based on statistically oriented clinical observation and a new focus on pathology based on local lesions – to come to the fore. But notwithstanding the increase in social distance between practitioners and their patients, and the shift in the balance of power in favour of the former, the conceptualisation of bodily processes developed by the early nineteenth-century French clinicians was nevertheless limited by the everyday exigencies of their occupational task, which restricted the clinical gaze to morbid events occurring within gross anatomical structures. However, as Jewson (1976: 237–238) has pointed out, the 'imagination and curiosity of laboratory scientists were not bound within these restrictions'.

Whereas hospital medicine reflected the interests and perceptions of clinicians, laboratory medicine was founded upon the worldview of the scientific research worker. A clear differentiation developed between the roles and careers of the research worker and those of the medical practitioner, with the former monopolising access to the laboratory facilities which rapidly became the essential means of production of new scientific knowledge. In Germany, university personnel who were likely to attain an international reputation for their contribution to knowledge rather than a local reputation for their pedagogic or therapeutic skills were sponsored by the Prussian state and this growing group of researchers developed a distinctive occupational ideology which emphasised the value of scientific work for its own sake, irrespective of any practical applications. And as the occupational activity of research workers increasingly took the form of the extension of scientific knowledge rather than the servicing of patients, the practical problems encountered in medical practice rapidly declined as a starting point for the investigations of scientific researchers (Jewson, 1976). Problems for investigation were increasingly defined not by the needs of sick patients, nor even by the perceptions of clinicians, but by problems and issues generated from within the nascent discipline of exercise physiology, where the focus was not on sick people but on the functioning of the *normal* body. This focus on the normal body is a point of central importance, and one to which we shall return on several occasions.

Hoberman (1992b: 237–239) has noted that during the second half of the nineteenth century, the German scientific establishment produced what may be called a 'latent sports physiology' which may be divided into five categories: muscle physiology; respiratory physiology; endocrine physiology; neuromotor physiology; and cardiac physiology. Given the significance of these scientific developments it is hardly surprising that they should be considered as important aspects of the early development of sports medicine. However, in tracing the development of modern sports medicine back to this period, there is a danger of overemphasising the continuities while failing to recognise the discontinuities in this developmental process. In this regard, it is important to note that the difference between contemporary sports medicine and the nascent discipline of sports medicine of the late nineteenth and early twentieth centuries lies not simply in the greater quantity of information which is now available, important though this undoubtedly is, but also in the fact that, in the earlier period, the orientations of the researchers and the problems they sought to resolve were also rather different from what they are now. This aspect of the changing structure of sports medicine has, perhaps, been brought out most clearly by Hoberman.

In describing the work of the early pioneers of sports medicine, Hoberman (1992b: 235–238, emphasis in original) emphasises that 'the investigation of human *athletic* potential was never a primary goal of the ethnographers and biological scientists who studied the human organism during this period', adding that 'the scientific marginality of sport during this period, its status as just one more potential application for physiological knowledge, cannot be sufficiently stressed'. He notes that a pioneering scientist like Nathan Zuntz 'did not do basic work on metabolism and muscle physiology, or put horses on his laboratory treadmill, to promote the fortunes of German athletics'.

In the late nineteenth century, the high-performance athlete was 'still a curiosity and not a charismatic figure at the centre of huge commercial enterprises like the Olympic Games' (Hoberman, 1992a: 6). Sport was considered as just one among a number of activities which were of interest to the physiologist and, as a source of interesting physiological data, sport occupied a relatively humble position within a much broader range of physical performances such as manual labour, military service, high altitude ballooning, singing and even coitus. As Hoberman (1992a: 6) has noted, the 'scientific marginality of sport during this period, and the general lack of interest in boosting (as opposed to investigating) athletic performance, has a quaintly premodern quality'.

The general absence among the pioneers of sports medicine of any interest in boosting athletic performance was a critical point of difference between the sports medicine of the late nineteenth and early twentieth centuries and the sports medicine of today. In relation to the former, Hoberman (1992a: 10) has pointed out that:

> the primary interest of these scientists was to discover the natural laws that regulated the functioning of the body. If they did not express an interest in applying science to the boosting of athletic performance it was in part because the scientific mysteries they found in the world of high-performance sport were already exciting enough.

Within the new mode of production of knowledge – laboratory medicine – the problems for investigation were defined not by the constraints to resolve short-term practical problems – and certainly not by a desire to improve athletic performance – but by the more fundamental scientific problems and issues generated from within the nascent discipline of physiology.

Not only is it the case that these scientists had little interest in boosting athletic performance, but it is also the case that some of the leading sports physicians of the period expressed concern about what they saw as the physiological dangers of sporting overexertion, not only for women – as Hargreaves (1994: 43) has noted, in the nineteenth century it was widely held, both within and outside the medical profession, that women 'were inherently emotional, cooperative and passive and therefore unsuited to take part in strenuous physical activities and competitive sports' (see also Pfister, 1990; Vertinsky, 1992) – but also for men and, for this reason, they actively opposed the search for new records in athletics. Particularly interesting in this respect was the career of Philippe Tissié, who was a contemporary and fellow countryman of Pierre de Coubertin and probably the most important sports physician of the *fin-de-siècle.* Although Tissié made some medical observations on a record-breaking long-distance cyclist, he actually disapproved of the high-performance sport of his era. Tissié did not share de Coubertin's view that breaking records was a central part of the athlete's task and he strongly opposed, because of what he saw as their medical dangers, the competitive sports which de Coubertin promoted. The conflict between the two came to a head in 1894 when, at the conference of the French Association for the Advancement of Science, Tissié successfully opposed de Coubertin's appeal for track-and-field events (Hoberman, 1992a: 80–84).

The early sports physicians, Hoberman suggests, saw 'sportive performances serving physiology as experimental data, rather than the other way round', with the emphasis being placed on the 'discovery of physiological laws rather than the application of these discoveries to athletic achievement'. In more recent years, however, the increased emphasis which has come to be placed on winning and on breaking records has dramatically changed the relationship between athletic performance and sports medicine. If, in the early years of the twentieth century, 'sport served the ends of science rather than the other way round', it is now the case that, in contrast to that earlier period, 'the modern outlook sees symbolic importance in the pursuit of the record performance, thereby putting physiology in the service of sport' (Hoberman, 1992a: ix, 78). This transition within the twentieth century was a process of great importance, and one which will be examined in more detail in later chapters.

The athletic body as the 'normal' body

Before concluding this section, it is necessary to elaborate a little on an important point which was touched on briefly earlier: the fact that while early physiological research was conducted on people involved in a wide variety of physical activities, including many non-sporting activities, all of those on whom the research was conducted were considered as normal, rather than as abnormal, examples of human physiology. In this regard, Heggie (2016) has correctly noted that even where data were collected from athletes who performed extraordinary athletic feats – for example, the English physiologist Frederick Pavy analysed the urine collected from the American long-distance pedestrian Edward Payson Weston during his attempt to walk 115 miles in London in 1876 – it was extremely rare for studies to be criticised because they used athletes as subjects. She also points out that when the American chemist Wilbur Atwater and his assistant, Charles Langworthy, published an extensive review of the existing literature on nutrition and diet in 1898, they divided the 3,800 studies in their review into those studying healthy and unhealthy bodies, in normal or abnormal conditions, but they did not consider it necessary to take into account whether the subjects were elite athletes or sedentary bank clerks. Elsewhere Heggie (2011: 52) notes that, even in the early twentieth century, the athletic body continued to be seen as 'the archetype of the normal body'.

The persistence of this view of the athletic body as the normal body had major implications for the development of sports medicine as a distinct branch of medical practice. In this regard, it should be noted that the persistence of the idea that the athletic body was the 'normal' body served to constrain the possibility of developing a new occupational group with a specialist body of knowledge or practice in this area, for since the athletic body was the normal body, it followed that athletes required no specialist medical care or support other than that provided for any other citizen. The development of sports medicine in its modern form, that is as a distinctive branch of medicine with its own specialist area of practice, was dependent on the articulation of a radically different perception of the athletic body: that the athletic body was *not* a normal body, that the athletes' physiology was *not* the same as the physiology of 'normal' people but that, on the contrary, the trained athlete is physiologically different from other, 'ordinary', people. This new view of the trained athlete was later to provide the central rationale for the development of a new specialist occupational group with its own distinctive forms of knowledge and practice, tailored specifically to the exceptional demands of this 'special' group of people. Such an occupational ideology began to emerge slowly in the twentieth century but, as we shall see later, it was not fully articulated until the period after the Second World War.

The provision of medical care to athletes

As we saw above, the work of laboratory-based scientists, particularly in Germany and France, considerably enhanced the understanding of human physiology from the middle years of the nineteenth century. However, it remains the case that, in most countries in the late nineteenth and early twentieth centuries, the *practice* of medicine by qualified doctors within the sporting arena was rare. In this section, we focus on the situation in Britain, while the situation in Germany, which played a critically important role in the early development of sports medicine, and specifically in the development of the formal institutional structure of sports medicine, is examined in the next chapter.

In Britain in the nineteenth and early twentieth centuries, athletes were inevitably sometimes injured as a result of their sporting activities and, as Cronin (2007: 26) has noted, they 'occasionally received some treatment'. Those most likely to receive any form of treatment were the small number of elite athletes, such as players involved in the newly professionalised sport of football. Those who provided this care constituted a highly diverse group of people, varying from those with little or no knowledge of medicine and the treatment of injuries to, very occasionally, qualified medical practitioners.

Carter (2009, 2012) has suggested that, following the introduction of professionalism into English football in 1885, a growing number of clubs began to employ 'trainers' of the kind who had earlier been employed by some boxers and pedestrians. The job of trainers included a number of off-field duties, including general day-to-day responsibility for the players, and fitness training as well as the treatment of injuries. In relation to the medical aspects of their role, Carter suggests that the origins of football trainers can be traced to unorthodox alternative medicine, and that their role developed largely outside of any medical regulatory framework. In this context, he suggests, 'they can be compared with irregular healers and alternative-unorthodox practitioners like bone-setters, herbalists and osteopaths'. Their methods and medical treatments were, he notes, the product of an oral and empirical tradition based on humoural theory – the general principles of which, as we saw earlier, had long since been undermined by developments in hospital and laboratory medicine – while treatment included the use of leeches, which had also been a central part of the therapeutic armoury of eighteenth century humoural medicine. Carter notes that football club trainers were not dependent on a doctor's patronage for a list of private patients, that there was no compunction on the part of trainers to develop closer links with orthodox medicine and that this allowed them to develop their own practices and methods in their own environment, away from medical supervision (Carter, 2009). It might be noted that the professionalisation of medical care within English football clubs was to be a long and painfully slow process; as late as 1953, and despite the very high incidence of injuries in professional football,[1] it was claimed that only 7 out of 92 Football League clubs had a physiotherapist (Carter, 2012).

In addition to club 'trainers', medical support was also available from a variety of other, largely unqualified, practitioners, including those offering massage. Massage was normally provided by 'rubbers', who would give a brisk rub down with a towel before and after competition, and they had frequently been used by pedestrians, boxers and rowers in the nineteenth century. Within a structure in which – unlike the highly complex world of modern sport – there was little specialised division of labour, the 'rubber' was frequently also the coach or trainer, team manager or promoter (Heggie, 2011: 47).

There was no professional massage organisation in Britain until the establishment of the Society of Trained Masseuses in 1894, a development which was prompted in part by a desire to differentiate between 'quacks' and those who had received some training, and which was stimulated, in part, by the 'Massage Scandal' of 1894, in which an article in the *British Medical Journal* about brothels masquerading as massage houses led to an investigation by police from Scotland Yard (Heggie, 2011: 46). However, it seems unlikely that the formation of the Society had any significant impact on the provision of medical care in football clubs or, indeed, most other sports. Full membership of the Society was only open to women until 1920, and Carter (2012) suggests that it was unlikely that football clubs, which were characterised by a highly masculine culture, would employ females, even qualified females, to massage their players while, for its part, the Society of Trained Masseuses showed little interest in the work of football and athletic trainers. Indeed, as Heggie (2011:47) notes, the Society had a rule that no 'general massage' should be given by its (female) members to men, and by 'general' was meant precisely the 'rubbing down' which was popular with players. In addition, the Society's rule that its members could only act under 'medical direction' would have effectively prohibited practice not just in professional football but in almost all sporting situations.

In addition to these sources of care there was during this period a large trade in what Carter (2012: 131) describes as 'quack remedies', as well as niche markets for massage liniments, herbal potions, patent pills and tonics which were directed, in part, at the sporting world, while Heggie (2011: 32) has pointed to the sale of food supplements, the manufacturer of one of which, Oxo, effectively sponsored the marathon at the 1908 London Olympics and was appointed by the British Olympic Association as 'official caterers'.

Footballers might occasionally be treated by qualified doctors, for example in the case of more serious injuries such as fractures, which would normally involve treatment at the local hospital. For professional players in the Manchester area, this might have involved treatment at Matlock House, which was established in the 1870s as an institute for general hydrotherapy but which gradually became popular with sportsmen, particularly professional footballers, and which became known as the Footballers' Hospital (Heggie, 2011: 61).

But for most athletes, treatment by qualified medical practitioners was rare. Cronin (2007: 25) has noted that 'few figures emerged in the … nineteenth-century annals of medicine who paid much attention to sport', that the few doctors who were involved in measuring and observing athletes 'represent only a small fraction of medical activity in nineteenth-century Britain' and that those who conducted such research were concerned with the bodily workings of athletes and not with the treatment of injuries. He argues that there is 'no identifiable sports medicine that comes into being during this period in Britain' and he asks: 'why did medicine fail to involve itself, at any active level, with sport?' (Cronin 2007: 23, 28). In order to answer this question, we need to examine contemporaneous developments in the medical profession.

In Britain in the second half of the nineteenth century, the medical profession was only just beginning to emerge from more than half a century of bitter and protracted infighting between different sections of the profession. This intra-professional conflict had its origins in major processes of structural change within the profession, particularly after 1800 (Waddington, 1975, 1984). The social and economic changes associated with the agricultural and industrial revolutions had not only expanded the demand for medical care, but had also created demands for a new type of medical care. Under the impact of these new patterns of demand, the traditional hierarchical division of labour between physicians, surgeons and apothecaries was rapidly breaking down and giving rise to the modern professional structure, based on the differentiation between general practitioners and hospital-based consultants. But while this traditional tripartite structure was crumbling, a new institutional structure appropriate to the newly emerging professional differentiation was slow in developing (Waddington, 1984). This resulted in a very confused situation, in which definitions of roles and statuses within the profession were very unclear, giving rise to continual and very acrimonious intra-professional disputes. The medical profession in the first half of the nineteenth century was, as Leake (1971: 70) has bluntly but accurately characterised it, 'a mess', and within this ambiguous and fluid situation, different types of practitioners 'jockeyed for positions of prestige and power'.

While many consultants enjoyed a market situation which was extremely lucrative, the incomes of general practitioners were much more modest and their incomes also suffered much more from the competition of unqualified practitioners than did those of consultants. In addition, the consultants effectively controlled both Royal Colleges, the most prestigious and powerful institutions within the profession. These differences in status, incomes and professional power gave rise to what proved to be an extraordinarily long and bitter campaign for medical reform on the part of general practitioners. The *Lancet,* under its founding editor, Thomas Wakley, was a consistent supporter of the general practitioners' campaign for reform, and the intensity of this campaign, and the vitriol which it generated, may be judged by the *Lancet's* description of hospital consultants, and those who controlled the Royal Colleges, as 'crafty, intriguing, corrupt, avaricious, cowardly, plundering, rapacious, soul-betraying, dirty-minded BATS' (*Lancet*, 1831-32, i: 2). The widely held picture of a profession as a harmonious and highly integrated community is not one which can readily be applied to the medical profession in the nineteenth century.

Some studies of the development of sports medicine in Britain from the nineteenth century have taken no regard of these conflicts and, after the usual brief obligatory reference to the 1858 Medical Act, have presented the process of professionalisation as relatively smooth (see, e.g., Carter, 2012). That it was nothing of the sort is indicated by the fact that the 1858 Medical Act, which established the General Medical Council and which gave the Council the responsibility of maintaining a register of qualified practitioners, was actually the 17th medical reform bill to have been introduced into Parliament since 1840, all previous bills having failed because of opposition from one section of the profession or the other. And although the 1858 Act is rightly seen as an important legislative landmark in the development of the modern medical profession in Britain, not least because it represented a first step towards a proper system of regulating medical practice on a national level, it by no means met all the demands of the general practitioners who continued to be concerned about what they considered as excessive competition both from without, and from within, the profession, and which many held to be the primary cause of their relatively modest incomes and status (Waddington, 1979, 1984, 1985).

Understanding the significance of these intra-professional problems is essential if we are to answer Cronin's question: why did medicine fail to involve itself, at any active level, with sport in the nineteenth century? In this regard, Cronin himself (2007: 31) correctly notes that while athletes were occasionally used by doctors for scientific research, 'the bulk of the profession – the general practitioner – was still engaged with a slower move towards respectability and societal respect, and for this group a relationship with sport was unimportant'. In short, treating the injuries of athletes offered neither a likely means of increasing one's practice income – there was of course no paid career structure for doctors who treated athletes – nor of improving the doctor's status either within the profession or the wider society. As we shall see, the relatively few doctors who did provide medical treatment to athletes did so not to enhance their medical careers or their incomes or status but, very often, simply because they had a personal involvement in – perhaps one might even say a passion for – playing and watching sport. It is, as we shall see, impossible to understand the development of sports medicine, not just in Britain but also in other countries, without taking into account this extra-scientific involvement in sport as an exciting and pleasurable leisure activity (Elias and Dunning, 1986). So who were the few doctors who provided medical support to athletes, and on what basis did they do so?

Carter (2012: 60) has noted that a strong sporting tradition developed among doctors in the nineteenth century, with Rugby Union being the sport of choice for many doctors. In this regard he notes that medical students at the London teaching hospitals had begun playing the game in the 1860s and that the United Hospitals Cup was established in 1874. Cronin (2007: 25) has also noted that there was a 'close relationship between medical colleges (especially in London) and active participation in playing sport'. That many doctors should have developed an interest in – and doubtless taken pleasure from – playing and/or watching sport is hardly surprising, for the modern forms of sporting competition which developed in the nineteenth century quickly proved enormously popular, especially with males, across all social classes (although there were then almost certainly, as there still are, marked social class differences in terms of the sports in which one chose to participate).[2] And it was from among this group of sports enthusiasts that the small number of doctors who provided medical care, most usually in the form of first aid, were largely drawn.

Cronin (2007: 25) has noted that

> any putative sports medicine, or at least a semblance of treatment in late nineteenth-century Britain, was reliant on a voluntaristic ethic of a small cohort of people. These would either be from the medical (interested doctors, often players) or the sporting field (players and coaches who favoured experimentation and self-treatment).

He adds that late nineteenth-century sports medicine, 'insofar as it existed at all, was the product of the interests of enthusiasts'. Heggie (2011) has similarly drawn attention to the importance of medically qualified 'enthusiasts', who were often (ex)sportsmen themselves or members of sports clubs, who actively sought out opportunities to work with athletes in providing first aid care on the field of play. And since there was no paid career structure for those who were involved in such 'work', they provided their services on a purely voluntary basis, as part of their personal involvement in and enthusiasm for sport. As we shall see, this personal, extra-scientific involvement in sport as an exciting and pleasurable activity is a central thread throughout the history of sports medicine; it was a key motivation among those involved in forming the early organisations representing practitioners in Germany, in the establishment of the Association Internationale Médico-Sportive in 1928 and in the establishment of national societies such as the British Association of Sport and Medicine in 1952, while recent research reveals that it remains, even today, as a key motivation for doctors to become involved in sports medicine (Waddington, Roderick and Parker, 1999; Malcolm, 2006). And as we shall see, this continuing thread is a key to understanding some important aspects of modern sports medicine as it developed in the twentieth century.

But how can we characterise the involvement of doctors in providing medical care to athletes in the late nineteenth and early twentieth centuries in Britain? Can this properly be described as the practice of sports medicine in any meaningful sense?

Perhaps the first point to note is that while there were a few doctors, largely sports enthusiasts, who offered voluntary first aid or other help to athletes, there is no evidence that, *as an occupational group*, the medical profession involved itself on the field of play by attending to or treating sportsmen. Cronin (2007: 26, 32) describes what he calls the 'apparent invisibility of sports medicine in the late nineteenth century' and suggests that 'the worlds of sport and medicine [were] largely separate in Victorian Britain'. Sport was, he suggests:

> never ideologically conceived in the nineteenth century as anything other than a manly pursuit that was underpinned by a moral code ... Injuries were therefore not seen as a problem requiring medical intervention and assistance but part of the rough and tumble of play. Real men were fearless and dealt with their injuries as best they could. They did not need to know scientifically how their bodies worked, and (especially for those working-class players on restricted incomes) they neither wanted nor sought the attention of doctors to treat their injuries.

Certainly it is the case that in the years before the First World War there was 'no critical mass of doctors who were identifiably allying themselves with sport as an area in which to practice' (Cronin, 2007: 25).

Heggie (2011: 25) takes a broadly similar position, noting that in the early decades of the twentieth century, 'there were no professional sports medicine organisations – no medical organisations dedicated to the needs of sport, and no sporting organisation with dedicated medical sub-committees ... Athletes appeared only rarely as the topics of (or guinea pigs in) papers in biomedical journals', while she suggests that the provision of medical services, even at national sporting events, was 'patchy' (Heggie, 2011: 33), a description which probably errs on the side of generosity. Outside of hospital care for more serious injuries such as fractures, qualified medical care for athletes was very limited and was dependent largely on volunteer doctors at the local level who were sports enthusiasts.

But the difference between the provision of medical care to athletes in the late nineteenth and early twentieth centuries and the practice of sports medicine today lies not simply in the much greater availability of care today, but also in the nature of the care which was offered. In this regard there are three central, interrelated issues. The first of these is the continued perception, in the earlier period, of the athletic body as 'normal', a view which was intimately linked to two other key issues: the perception and treatment of sports injuries as 'normal', rather than as sports-specific, and the relative lack of concern with performance enhancement.

Heggie (2011: 30) has suggested that there are three dimensions of the practice of sports medicine, each with specific aims: (i) treatment, much of which is essentially first aid; (ii) enhancement, that is, the use of biomedical and biochemical knowledge to alter and improve performance; and (iii) prevention, particularly the prevention of injury. She notes that between 1900 and 1927, basic treatment certainly occurred, whether in the form of first aid or hospital treatment for more serious injuries, but that enhancement and prevention are harder to locate. Cronin (2007: 26–27) has similarly noted that even those doctors with an interest in sport 'were not overly concerned … with offering sports medicine to sportsmen as something that could be consumed as a way of improving their performance, or ensuring they return to full fitness in as quick a time as possible'. In relation to enhancement, Heggie points out that while athletic training manuals contained advice (which sometimes claimed to be based on scientific research) which sought to bring athletes to peak condition for competition, they sought to do so simply by ensuring the athlete was in good health, thus permitting them to reach their natural limits, rather than to expand them. Such 'enhancement' as there was took place within the confines of the body's normal abilities and limits, and Heggie (2011: 28–29) correctly notes that 'it is not until well into the twentieth century that sports doctors seriously begin to talk about manufacturing and creating supernormal performances and enhanced physiques'.

If the athletic body continued to be seen as normal, injuries received within the sporting context also continued to be seen, by athletes and doctors alike, like any other injury, so that the sporting context of the injury was not seen as relevant to either the aetiology or the treatment of the injury. As Cronin (2007: 25) has noted:

> Injuries to the sporting body were not conceived, once they had happened, as sporting injuries requiring specialist sports medicine care. The treatment of such injuries … if undertaken at all, was driven more by the need of the athlete to return to his paid employment than any concerns about restoring full athletic or match fitness. The failure of athletes to see their injuries as sports specific, was assisted by a lack of awareness amongst the medical profession that they should view sports injuries, and their treatment, as a valid practice or specialization.

A good example is provided by the treatment received in hospital by footballers who had the misfortune to fracture a leg; such players would be treated in much the same way as any other patient with a fractured limb and the techniques used would not be techniques which had been developed specifically with a view to treating players with special requirements, for example in relation to a rapid return to play and match fitness – both of which are, of course, major constraints on both doctors and their athlete-patients in the modern practice of sports medicine (Waddington, Roderick and Parker, 1999; Waddington, 2000, 2012; Roderick, Waddington and Parker, 2000) – but techniques which had been developed in the context of treating the much more common fractures which occurred in industrial, agricultural and vehicle accidents. For the most part athletes asked for, and received, no special treatment because they did not conceptualise themselves as, and were not conceptualised by doctors as, special, that is, as a distinctive group of patients. A radical medical reconceptualisation of athletes was required before a clear basis could be constructed for the development of sports medicine as a specialist branch of practice. This is one reason, among others, why the provision of medical care to athletes in the late nineteenth and early twentieth centuries may perhaps be most accurately described not as the practice of sports medicine, but as the application of general medical knowledge to the athlete or, more simply, as medicine applied to sport.

But if there were several characteristics which distinguish modern sports medicine from its earlier predecessors, there was one important characteristic which they had in common: a central focus on elite-level sport. We noted earlier that Heggie described medical services in the early twentieth century at local and even national sporting events as 'patchy', but she adds that this patchy provision was 'outclassed by the provision at international level'. Medical provision at the London Olympics of 1908 followed the pattern of previous and subsequent Olympics, with voluntary medical services provided by St John Ambulance while competing teams either brought their own medical staff or bought the services of local doctors and hospitals. The marathon was the subject of particular medical interest, with seven 'medical attendants and examiners', six of whom held the title 'Dr', while medical professionals, appointed by the British Olympic Association, also patrolled the course (Heggie, 2011: 34). The Olympics represented then, as now, the highest level of international sporting competition, and this focus on elite level competitive sport was to remain a central feature of modern sports medicine as it developed in the twentieth century and one which, as we shall see, helped to steer the development of sports medicine in a particular direction.

Notes

1 One study found that the overall risk of injury in professional football in England was 1,000 times higher than the risk of injury in other occupations normally regarded as high risk, such as construction and mining (Hawkins and Fuller, 1999).

2 For an outline of the current situation in relation to class and sporting participation in Britain, see Waddington (2020).

References

Carter, N. (2009), The rise and fall of the magic sponge: medicine and the transformation of the football trainer, *Social History of Medicine*, 23 (2), 261–279.

Carter, N. (2012), *Medicine, Sport and the Body: A Historical Perspective*, London, Bloomsbury.

Cronin, M, (2007), Not taking the medicine: sportsmen and doctors in late nineteenth-century Britain, *Journal of Sport History*, 34 (1), 23–35.

Dunning, E. (1986), The dynamics of modern sports: notes on achievement-striving and the social significance of sport, in N. Elias and E. Dunning (eds), *Quest for Excitement: Sport and Leisure in the Civilizing Process*, Oxford, Blackwell, 205–223.

Elias, N. and Dunning, E. (1986), *Quest for Excitement: Sport and Leisure in the Civilizing Process*, Oxford, Blackwell.

Hawkins, R. D. and Fuller, C. W. (1999), A prospective epidemiological study of injuries in four English professional football clubs, *British Journal of Sporst Medicine*, 33, 196–203.

Hargreaves, J. (1994), *Sporting Females: Critical Issues in the History and Sociology of Women's Sports*, London, Routledge.

Heggie, V. (2011), *A History of British Sports Medicine*, Manchester, Manchester University Press.

Heggie, V. (2016), Bodies, sport and science in the nineteenth century, *Past and Present*, 231(1), 169–200.

Hoberman. J. (1992a), *Mortal Engines: The Science of Performance and the Dehumanization of Sport,* New York, Free Press.

Hoberman, J. (1992b), The early development of sports medicine in Germany, in J. W. Berryman and R. J. Park (eds), *Sport and Exercise Science: Essays in the History of Sports Medicine*, Urbana and Chicago, University of Illinois Press, 233–282.

Jewson, N. (1976), The disappearance of the sick-man from medical cosmology 1770–1870, *Sociology*, 10, 225–244.

Leake, C. D. (1971), Percival's Medical Ethics: promise and problems, *California Medical*, 114, 68–70.

Malcolm, D. (2006), Sports medicine: a very peculiar practice? in S. Loland, B.Skirstad and I. Waddington (eds), *Pain and Injury in Sport: Social and Ethical Analysis,* Oxon, Routledge, 165–181.

Pfister, G. (1990), The medical discourse on female physical culture in Germany in the 19th and early 20th centuries, *Journal of Sport History*, 17 (2), 183–198.

Roderick, M., Waddington, I. and Parker, G. (2000), Playing hurt: managing injuries in English professional football, *International Review for the Sociology of Sport*, 35 (2), 165–180.

Vertinsky, P. (1992), Exercise, physical capability, and the eternally wounded woman in late nineteenth-century North America, in J. W. Berryman and R. J. Park (eds), *Sport and Exercise Medicine: Essays in the History of Sports Medicine*, Urbana and Chicago, University of Illinois Press, 183–211.

Waddington, I. (1975), The development of medical ethics: a sociological analysis, *Medical History*, 19 (1), 36–51.

Waddington, I. (1979), Competition and monopoly in a profession: the campaign for medical registration in Britain, *Amsterdams Sociologisch Tijdschrift*, 6 (2), 288–321.

Waddington, I. (1984), *The Medical Profession in the Industrial Revolution*, Dublin, Gill and Macmillan.

Waddington, I. (1985), Medicine, the market and professional autonomy: some aspects of the professionalization of medicine, in W. Conza and J. Kocka (eds), *Bildungsbürgertum im 19. Jahrhundert*, Stuttgart, Klett-Cotta, 388–416.

Waddington, I. (2000), *Sport, Health and Drugs*, London, Spon.

Waddington, I. (2012), Sports medicine, client control and the limits of professional autonomy, in D. Malcolm and P. Safai (eds), *The Social Organization of Sports Medicine: Critical Socio-Cultural Perspectives,* New York, Routledge, 204–226.

Waddington, I. (2020), Sport and Welfare in Britain, in N. Porro, S. Martelli and A. Testa (eds), *Sport, Welfare and Social Policy in the European Union*, London, Routledge, 99–109.

Waddington, I., Roderick, M. and Parker, G. (1999), *Managing Injuries in Professional Football: A Study of the Roles of the Club Doctor and Physiotherapist*, Leicester, Centre for Research into Sport and Society, University of Leicester.

4 The early movement towards the institutionalisation of sports medicine

German scientists and medical practitioners played an important part in the early development of sports medicine. As we saw in the previous chapter, German universities played a leading role in the development of laboratory medicine, and by the early twentieth century, Germany was a leading nation not only in terms of exercise physiology but also in terms of medicine and science more generally (Pfister, 2011: 280; Krüger, 2015: 334). Specifically in relation to the development of sports medicine, Germany recorded a number of significant 'firsts'. The term 'sports physician' (*Sportarzt*) was first used in 1904 by Arthur Mallwitz, a very prominent sports physician during the early decades of the twentieth century who was centrally involved not only in the establishment of the first association of sports physicians in Germany but also in the establishment in 1928 of the Association Internationale Médico-Sportive (AIMS). The first official congress of sports physicians took place in Oberhof in 1912, while the first university lecture course in sports medicine was given by Mallwitz and the surgeon August Bier in 1919. The world's first sports college, which included a sports medicine curriculum, was founded in Berlin in 1920. In the 1920s Germany was the only country in the world with an association of sports doctors, which was established in 1924 following the second German Sports Physicians' Congress, held earlier that year. From 1925, the first sports medicine journal, *Der Sportarzt/Sportärztliche Mitteilungen* [The Sports Physician/Sports Medical Bulletin], was published as a supplement to *Klinische Wochenschrift* [Clinical Weekly Review]. The first book to use the term 'sports medicine' in its title was a German book, Dr Herbert Herxheimer's *Grundriss der Sportsmedizin*, published in 1933, a full three decades before the publication of the first book in English to use the term in its title, J. G. P. Williams's *Sports Medicine*, published in 1962 (Ryan, 1989; Pfister, 2011; Krüger, 2015; Hoberman, 1992a, 1992b). It is these institutional developments within sports medicine which are the focus of this chapter.

But before we examine these institutional developments, it is important to say a few words about the early use of the term *Sportarzt*. As Asa Briggs long ago noted in his classic essay, *The language of class in early nineteenth century England*, a concern with the origins and usage of such terms is 'not simply an academic exercise in semantics'. In this regard, he suggested that 'the concept of "social" class, with all its attendant terminology was a product of the large-scale economic and social changes of the late eighteenth and early nineteenth

DOI: 10.4324/9781003563921-6

centuries'. The change in nomenclature in this period, which involved a shift away from the pre-industrial language of 'ranks', 'orders' or 'interests' and towards the language of social class, 'reflected a basic change not only in men's (sic) ways of viewing society but in society itself'. Put succinctly it is important to understand the relationship between words and social changes (Briggs, 1960: 43–44).

As in the case of the use of the term 'class' to describe the newly emerging pattern of social divisions and inequalities associated with the development of industrial capitalism in England, so too the use of the term *Sportarzt* reflected both the incipient development of, and the first recognition of, a newly emerging type of doctor, and the fact that the term was first used in Germany is indicative of the relatively early development of aspects of sports medicine in that country. However, the introduction and early use of the word *Sportarzt* should not be taken as an indication that in the early decades of the twentieth-century sports medicine had emerged in anything like the specialised discipline that we know today. The comparison with the use of the term 'class' is again instructive here. Royle (1987: 84) has noted that the first uses of the terms 'middle class' and 'working class' appear to date from 1766 and 1789, respectively, that is at a time when England was still mainly a rural society and when industrial production – and the modern class structure based on the industrial mode of production – was still very much in its infancy. In much the same way, it might be said that the early use of the term *Sportarzt* represented not the establishment of a new subdiscipline within medicine, but rather the first signs of recognition – perhaps the first signs of a change in the self-perception of a few doctors – that their interest in sport might lead them in a potentially new direction of practice.

But this new direction of practice was, even in Germany, still in its infancy. In the 1920s, there was widespread agreement, even among those who were members of the newly formed association of sports physicians, that sports medicine should not become a separate medical discipline. Dr Walter Schnell, the president of the association, pointed out in 1927 that, on a purely practical level, physicians specialising in sports medicine would simply have difficulty making a living, while two years previously he had pointed to a more fundamental problem, namely that the 'specific nature of the sports medical consultation does not involve the development of a special method, but rather the application of established medical science of a specific area' (Schnell, 1925, cited in Hoberman, 1992b: 241). In other words, there was no clear scientific basis, nor as yet any clearly articulated occupational ideology, which could provide a rationalisation for sports medicine as a distinct branch of practice. And if there was no clear scientific rationale or occupational ideology to justify the establishment of sports medicine as a separate branch of practice, it is also the case that at a practical level, medical support to athletes remained relatively scarce on the ground; Pfister (2011: 284) has noted that before World War II 'there was no systematic medical supervision, even for Olympic sportsmen and women'. But let us examine the other key institutional developments within Germany.

The early institutionalisation of sports medicine in Germany

For much of the nineteenth century, the predominant form of physical culture had been German gymnastics (*Turnen*), a system of pedagogic exercises developed at the time of the Napoleonic Wars by Friedrich Ludwig Jahn, the 'father of German gymnastics', who linked *Turnen* with what Reicher (2020: 213) has called 'fierce German nationalism'. The nationalistic message of those who supported *Turnen* was clear: 'that gymnastics contribute to the *Volksgesundheit* – the health of the people – which is … a precondition for the soundness of the German nation and its strength or power, compared to other people and nations' (Krüger, 2015: 337). But Jahn's idea of *Turnen* went far beyond physical exercise and a concern with physical health. Pfister (2003: 65) has noted that the concepts of *Volk, Volkstum and Volkserziehung*, signifying the German people, their common heritage and a public education based on this common heritage, 'were key words in Jahn's *Turnen*'. She adds that *Turnen* 'was more than merely physical exercise, and important ingredients were patriotic speeches, traditional songs, celebrations held to commemorate important events of German history and excursions intended to give young men an opportunity of getting to know and to love their fatherland'.

The introduction of 'English' sports into Germany in the late nineteenth century gave a renewed impetus to the *Turnen* movement, which became a symbol of German 'cultural uniqueness' and an expression of German 'national character' (Reicher, 2020: 215). Supporters of *Turnen* were opposed to modern sport which they saw as a foreign (primarily English) import. They argued that sport was characterised by an obsession with competition and breaking records, while they also drew upon a variety of nationalistic, racial and ethnic arguments to justify their opposition. The result of these tensions was a power struggle fought out in the first sports medicine associations in the early twentieth century between physicians who supported *Turnen* and those who supported modern competitive sports. The outcome of that power struggle was, as we shall see below, to prove of major importance for the subsequent development of sports medicine, not only in Germany but also in the wider world.

The First International Hygiene Exhibition, held in Dresden in 1911, was designed to provide information to the general public about health and healthcare issues, but the exhibition also included a section devoted to sports and games. The focus was not on sporting performance but on both the beneficial and negative effects of exercise on health. In relation to the latter, Pfister (2011: 275) has noted that the increasing popularity of modern sports had 'added to concerns about the negative effects of sport, and warnings were issued in particular about excessive strain and physical exertion'. It may well be the case that these warnings expressed the concerns of those doctors who were sympathetic to *Turnen*, many of whom were opposed to modern sport, which they saw as an overspecialised form of physical culture which was stressful and harmful to health.

In the following year, a group of physicians, many of whom had been involved in the organisation of the 1911 Hygiene Exhibition, founded the *Vereinigung zur wissenschaftlichen Erforschung des Sports und der Leibesubüngen* (Association for the Scientific Research of Sport and Physical Exercises), based in Berlin. Their central concern was with sport and exercise as a means of promoting public health, rather than with high-level competitive sport. One of the central figures involved in the establishment of the Berlin Association, and also of the earlier International Hygiene Exhibition, was Georg Friedrich Nicolai, a professor at the Charité Hospital in Berlin, who held that while games and exercise could help to promote public health, elite sport was a 'luxury' which should be of no interest to physicians (Pfister, 2011: 2176). His ideas about sport (and also his ideas about war – he was a pacifist) were attacked by most of his colleagues, most notably by Arthur Mallwitz, who had himself been an elite athlete – he had represented Germany in several events in the 1906 Intercalated Games in Athens and again in the London summer Olympics of 1908 (www.olympedia.org) – and who also later joined the Nazi party. These conflicts represented the beginnings of a power struggle for control of the emerging institutions of sports medicine and, in particular, a struggle to define the nature of sports medicine and its position in relation to modern high-level competitive sport.

In the same year that the Berlin Association was formed, the first official German congress of sports physicians was held at a hotel in Oberhof, and during the congress discussions took place which led to the formation in September 1912 of the *Deutsche Reichskomitee für die wissenschaftliche Erforschung des Sports und der Leibesübungen* (German Committee for the Scientific Research of Sport and Exercise). The vice-president of the Berlin Association, Friedrich Kraus, was elected as its first chairman and, perhaps not surprisingly given their radically different views of the nature and significance of sport, the early period of the new committee was overshadowed by conflicting interests and controversies between the Berlin association and the *Reichskomitee*, as well as between Nicolai and Mallwitz (Pfister, 2011: 277).

The position of Mallwitz and those whose interest was in high-level competitive sport was considerably strengthened by the growing influence of the *Deutscher Reichsausschuss für Olympische Spiele* (German Olympic Committee), which became an increasingly important player in sports research as part of the preparations for the 1916 Olympic Games, which were scheduled to be held in Berlin. Pfister (2011: 277) has noted that the German Olympic Committee, 'as well as Mallwitz and many others, emphasised the significance of sports science for performance enhancement, whereas Nicolai and the Berlin Association placed sport and sports medicine in the public health discourses'. In 1914, the German Olympic Committee accepted Mallwitz's proposal to establish a research facility on the outskirts of Berlin with a focus on sporting targets, sporting performance and training methods, a decision which marked a 'significant paradigm shift in sports science' (Pfister, 2011: 277). The proposed 1916 Olympics were of course cancelled because of the war, but even during the war the German Olympic Committee set up a scientific research committee charged with the task of studying issues relating to improving athletic performance (Pfister, 2011: 177).

Following the war, Germany became the first country to establish a professional association of sports physicians when in 1924, at a conference attended by

300 doctors and 200 representatives of various administrative bodies, a decision was taken to form the *Deutscher Ärztebund zur Förderung der Leibesübungen* [German Medical Association for the Advancement of Physical Activities – DÄB]. Mallwitz was elected as vice-chair of the DÄB and from an initial membership of 62 in 1924, membership grew to 2,289 in 1927 and to over 3,000 in 1933 (Pfister, 2011: 278–279).

The members of the DÄB came from a variety of medical specialities and this was reflected in the variety of research interests, which included health education, sports injuries and studies of performance and performance improvement in sport. However, Pfister (2011: 285) notes that gradually, 'medical discourse began to focus on the question of how performance in sport might be improved'. By the late 1920s, the shifting balance of power within the DÄB in favour of supporters of modern high-level competitive sport was clear, and this shifting balance of power reflected wider changes in playing and watching sports in German society. Although advocates of *Turnen* continued their resistance to modern sport until well into the 1920s, there was a marked decline in support for nationalistic German gymnastics from the 1920s (Reicher, 2020). *Turnen* had always been largely a bourgeois activity, while the nobility – which remained very powerful in Germany until the First World War – and the Kaiser had quickly adopted modern sports, with the Kaiser even providing money to German athletes to support their participation in the 1896 Athens Olympics. And while many supporters of *Turnen* had strongly opposed working-class membership of gymnastic associations, the new sports, especially football and Olympic sports, grew rapidly in popularity, with a widespread appeal across the social classes (Reicher, 2020). The result was that, by the 1920s, instead of the traditional German exercises, a growing number of *Turnen* clubs began to offer track and field sports, while even some forms of gymnastics, for example gymnastics on apparatus, became increasingly oriented towards performance and competition (Pfister, 2003: 84).

Within the DÄB, this shift towards high-level competitive sport and towards questions related to improving performance was expressed in a variety of ways. Mallwitz was himself a pioneer in this respect. The Organizing Committee of the 1896 Athens Olympic Games had agreed that Mallwitz and two other German physicians should be allowed to examine competing athletes with respect to their anatomical and anthropometric characteristics as well as heart function and, over the whole period from 1891 to 1906, Mallwitz and his colleagues examined more than 100 elite athletes (Berg and König 2002: 3). In 1908 Mallwitz had defended his dissertation on the effects of high-performance sport on the human organism, in which he drew upon his own experience as an elite athlete to suggest that his success in the 1906 Intercalated Games in Athens, and that of a German teammate, had confirmed another scientist's prognostications since their relatively small hearts had not precluded successful performances (Hoberman 1992b: 241).

In the 1920s, anthropometric measurements of the kind which Mallwitz had undertaken some years earlier became a common theme of research, with a catalyst in this area being the work of Wilhelm Kohlrausch who had suggested that particular types of body structure and temperament were associated with particular types of sporting events; Hoberman (1992: 251) has correctly noted that the application of this 'constitutional theory' to sport may be seen as an early example of what later became known as 'aptitude testing'. The 1920s also saw the development, in close cooperation with sports physicians, of biomechanics which, among other things, used film of athletes in motion to see how movements might be optimised. Other areas of study included the body's expenditure of energy in the course of physical exertion, the role of diet in performance and any measures which it was thought might enhance performance, from massage to infra-red lamps and the use of 'artificial stimulants' (Pfister, 2011: 286).

The search for enhanced performance also encompassed the use of pharmacological products. In the interwar period, the use of drugs in German sport was already widespread and widely known (Hoberman, 1992a: 134). In his address to the annual meeting of the German Swimming Association in 1933, Professor Otto Riesser, of the University of Breslau, stated that 'sportive competitions are often more a matter of doping than of training'. He held that physicians were not without blame for this situation, 'in part because they are prescribing strong drugs for the purpose of doping which are not available to athletes without prescriptions' (cited in Hoberman, 1992a: 131–132). Those involved in the use of pharmacological products included some of the most celebrated sports physicians in Germany. For example, one of the physicians whom Riesser might have had in mind was Dr Martin Brustmann, who was one of the physicians who had helped Mallwitz with the examination of athletes at the 1896 Athens Olympic Games. In 1912 he published a book on training for track and field athletes, but he also became well-known for using performance-enhancing drugs, being described in a popular magazine as 'an expert in the field of pharmaceutical "fuels for will-power"' (Reinold and Meier, 2012: 9). Brustmann went on to enjoy a long and successful career coaching top national and international athletes but is probably most remembered for his part in the 'Brustmann affair' of 1952, in which he administered pills containing male sex hormones to a German rowing crew; significantly this incident became a national scandal not because he had administered hormone pills with a view to enhancing performance, but because the pills appear to have had the reverse effect, of reducing performance, so that Brustmann was accused of 'negative doping', more normally associated with animal sports (Reinold and Meier, 2012).

Herbert Herxheimer, author of the much-cited *Grundriss der Sportsmedizin*, published in 1933, was also involved in experiments with performance-enhancing drugs (Reinold and Meier, 2012: 5). In 1922, he had already claimed that the commercial product Recresal (primary sodium phosphate) produced a significant increase in physical fitness. Hoberman has suggested that more interesting than Herxheimer's endorsement of the product, however, 'are the verbal gymnastics that follow'. Herxheimer suggested that, with the approach of a new sports season, the aspiring athlete would need to take phosphates. Without mentioning the word 'doping', he went on to describe the use of phosphates as an ergogenic 'aid' (*Hilfe*) which, he argued, was quite different from the many 'stimulants' in use, since it merely 'supported' basic physiological processes (Hoberman, 1992a: 134).

Other sports physicians engaged in similar 'verbal gymnastics'. For example, W. Poppelreuter, a professor of medicine in Bonn, pointed to the significance of Recresal for athletic performance, but he argued that this was a 'normal hygienic procedure' which should not be equated with the use of strychnine or cocaine and other types of 'doping'. Poppelreuter suggested that sport had a key role to play in the rational use of human nutrients, whether they are considered natural or artificial and, like Herxheimer, he insisted that 'doping', which he considered harmful, should be sharply distinguished from the use of substances that 'support' basic physiological systems (Hoberman, 1992a: 135).

A second argument which was used by German sports physicians to differentiate their provision of 'support' from 'doping' centred on the temporal dimension, that is the difference between short and longer-term effects of pharmacological products on athletes. Thus a distinction was drawn between a pharmacological product taken just before competition to boost performance and a product taken in training as part of longer-term preparation for competition (Hoberman, 1992a: 141). In this, as in many other aspects of sports medicine, Germany led the way; as we shall see later, the 'verbal gymnastics' practised by German sports physicians – both the argument that a distinction should be made between pharmacological products which enhanced performance by 'supporting' physiological systems and those which enhanced performance by 'doping', as well as the temporal differentiation between 'doping' and 'preparation' – were also widely used by French sports physicians from the 1950s.

If the early years of the institutionalisation of sports medicine in Germany had been marked by a power struggle – Pfister (2003: 76) refers to 'notorious conflicts' – between advocates of *Turnen*, who located exercise primarily within a (nationalistic) public health context, and supporters of competitive high-performance sport, it is clear that by the late 1920s and early 1930s, the balance of power had shifted decisively in favour of the latter. Pfister (2011: 287) has noted that by this time there had been a shift not only towards competitive elite sport but 'toward questions of performance and performance enhancement'. By the 1930s, sports medicine in Germany had a clear focus on elite-level competitive sport with a growing emphasis on performance enhancement. It may be argued that it was in this period that the foundations of what became the (in)famous high-performance sports medicine systems of both East and West Germany in the 1970s and 1980s were laid. And the increasingly close association between sports medicine and high-level competitive sport was further consolidated in an institutional development of considerable importance: the formation at the 1928 Winter Olympic Games of the Association Internationale Médico-Sportive (AIMS), which in 1934 became the Fédération Internationale de Médecine Sportive (FIMS).

The establishment of FIMS

Heggie (2011: 65) has noted that the year 1928 'would stand out in any sports medicine chronography'. In Germany in that year, full-time chairs in sports medicine were established in universities in Hamburg and Leipzig, while in the UK the British Olympic Association appointed its first official Medical Officer and Adolphe Abrahams, who had long been the unofficial Olympic team doctor, undertook a physiological survey of British Olympic competitors. But without question the most important landmark in the development of modern sports medicine in that year was the establishment of AIMS, later FIMS.

Given the relatively high level of development of sports medicine in Germany, it is not perhaps surprising that German sports physicians played a central role in the establishment of the first international association of sports doctors. Neither is it perhaps surprising that some of the central features of sports medicine, as it was emerging in Germany, were institutionalised within the structure of FIMS.

In February 1928, on the occasion of the second Winter Olympics at St Moritz, Switzerland, a meeting of doctors attending those Olympic Games was held at the invitation of Dr Wilhelm Knoll and the Swiss Olympic Committee. At that meeting, at which the French physiologist André Latarjet emphasised the contribution of German doctors to the development of sports medicine, a decision was taken to establish the Association Internationale Médico-Sportive (AIMS). Many competitors at those Winter Olympics were medically examined before and after their performance. Siemens installed X-ray equipment without charge and the Swiss Red Cross provided a number of barracks in which medical examinations were carried out. Competitors were anthropologically examined, an X-ray was taken of their hearts and their blood circulation and metabolism were checked. Six months later, at the Summer Olympic Games in Amsterdam, AIMS held its first International Conference of Sports Medicine and, at those Games, a larger programme of research was carried out on competing athletes with the twin aims of gaining a better understanding of athletes' training conditions and identifying any potential problems that could arise from participation in high-level sports. Research was carried out on anthropometry, strength measurements, reaction times and recovery after fatigue, blood, sweat and urine samples were analysed, and competitors were given a general medical examination (https://medicosport.eu/en/history/history1928.html). Following the AIMS research programme at the Summer Olympics in 1928, the Olympic Games became the regular site of medical research into the bodies of elite athletes.

Little is known about most of the doctors who attended the initial meeting of AIMS at St Moritz, but it is known that the 33 (or in some reports 50) doctors who attended came from eleven countries. Germany was strongly represented, with no fewer than 12 German doctors attending. Knoll was the first President. Although he was Swiss, Knoll had close ties with Germany, having received part of his medical education in Germany and having worked in Tübingen; he was later appointed to a post in Hamburg and in 1933 became a member of the Nazi Party. Arthur Mallwitz was the first Secretary General.

It is important to emphasise that it was no accident that the establishment of AIMS took place at an Olympic Games. We noted in Chapter 2 that in the late nineteenth century, medical practitioners had largely withdrawn their earlier interest in exercise as a health-promoting activity for the general population and had ceded the management and control of this area of activity to educationalists, sports masters and coaches in schools and colleges. In Chapter 3, we noted that in England during the latter part of the nineteenth and early twentieth centuries, the relatively few doctors with an interest in sports medicine had focused their medical assistance on professional and elite-level competitive sport. And we noted earlier that in Germany, those who favoured a focus on high-performance competitive sport had, with the support of the German Olympic Committee, emerged by the late 1920s as victorious in the power struggle against those who supported the nationalistic *Turnen* movement, and who had opposed high-level competitive sport and favoured programmes of largely non-competitive exercise linked with public health.

The establishment of AIMS at the Winter Olympics, together with the follow-up conference and programme of research on elite athletes at the Summer Olympics in Amsterdam, *effectively consolidated at the international level this developing relationship between sports medicine and elite level competitive sport.* Then, as now, the Olympic Games represented the highest level of international sport, and the establishment of AIMS at the Olympic Games not only identified sports medicine with competitive sport, but with competitive sport at the very highest level. AIMS was, in effect, born under the umbrella of the Olympic Games, and the strong association between FIMS and the Olympic Games is symbolised in the five Olympic rings which are still today incorporated in the flag and logo of FIMS. With the establishment of AIMS, sports medicine was unambiguously identified as an adjunct to high-level sport, rather than as an element of public health.

The establishment of AIMS at the 1928 Winter Olympics thus defined what was to be the basis of the subsequent development of sports medicine for the next 60 years: an almost exclusive focus on competitive athletes in high-performance, elite-level sport. The importance of this point can hardly be overstated; it is absolutely central to understanding the growing involvement of sports physicians in enhancing sporting performance and the growing centrality of enhancing performance as a raison d'être of sports medicine, especially from the 1950s.

References

Berg, A. and König, D (2002), History of sports medicine in Germany with special reference to the University of Freiburg, *European Journal of Sport Science*, 2 (4), 1–7.

Briggs, A. (1960), The language of 'class' in early nineteenth century England, in A. Briggs and J. Saville (eds), *Essays in Labour History*, London, Palgrave Macmillan, 43–73.

Heggie, V. (2011), *A History of British Sports Medicine*, Manchester, Manchester University Press.

Hoberman. J. (1992a), *Mortal Engines*, New York, The Free Press.

Hoberman, J. (1992b), The early development of sports medicine in Germany, in J. W. Berryman and R. J. Park (eds), *Sport and Exercise Science: Essays in the History of Sports Medicine*, Urbana and Chicago, University of Illinois Press, 233–282.

Krüger, M. (2015), History of sport medicine in Germany. Some preliminary reflections on a complex research project, *Historical Social Research*, 40 (4), 331–349.

Pfister, G. (2003), Cultural confrontations: German *Turnen*, Swedish gymnastics and English sport – European diversity in physical activities from a historical perspective, *Culture, Sport, Society*, 6 (1), 61–91.

Pfister, G. (2011), 'Sports' medicine in Germany and its struggle for professional status, *Canadian Bulletin of Medical History*, 28 (2), 271–292.
Reicher, D. (2020), Nationalistic German gymnastic movements and modern sports. Culture between identity and habitus, *Historical Social Research/Historische Sozialforschung*, 45 (2), special edition Emotion, Authority, and National Character, 207–225.
Reinold, M. and Meier, H. E. (2012), Difficult adaptations to innovations in performance enhancement: 'Dr Brustmann's power pills' and anti-doping in German post-war sport, *Sport in History*, 1–31.
Royle, E. (1987), *Modern Britain: A Social History 1750–1997*, London, Arnold.
Ryan, A. J. (1989), Sports Medicine in the World Today, in A. J. Ryan and F. L. Allman, Jr, *Sports Medicine*, 2nd edn, San Diego, Academic Press.
Schnell, W. (1925), Der Sportartz, *Die Leibesübungen.*

5 The physician-athlete and the development of sports medicine

In the previous chapter we described some of the major institutional developments within sports medicine in early twentieth century Germany. In addition to these institutional developments, there was one other aspect of the early development of sports medicine which is of particular significance for understanding its subsequent pattern of development. In this regard, Hoberman has noted that many sports physicians were, or had been, athletes and he uses the concept of the physician-athlete to draw attention to the fact that German sports medicine 'originated … among physicians with a personal interest in sport' (Hoberman, 1992: 239). Hoberman (1992: 240) appears to have been the first – and until now the only – scholar to use the label 'physician-athlete', but he leaves the concept of the physician-athlete undeveloped. We suggest that the concept, if carefully unpacked, has considerable heuristic value and that it has much wider applicability than to just the German situation in the early twentieth century. In this regard, it is important to emphasise that the concept of the physician-athlete does not indicate that the doctor treats athletes, but that very frequently the doctor *is* an athlete or ex-athlete. In this regard, we would suggest that while the label 'sports physician' is an occupational title which tells us what the doctor does, the label physician-athlete is a more personal label which tells us something about *who the doctor is*.

Hoberman (1992: 240) has noted that, in the early decades of the twentieth century, 'German sports physicians tended to agree that they should be active or former athletes'. We have already noted that, among prominent sports physicians, Arthur Mallwitz, perhaps the leading figure in the development of sports medicine in Germany in the early nineteenth century, was also an Olympic athlete. Martin Brustmann who, as we noted earlier, was one of the physicians who worked with Mallwitz in the examination of athletes at the 1896 Athens Olympic Games, was, like Mallwitz, also an elite athlete. With Mallwitz, he represented Germany in the Intercalated Games in Athens in 1906 and he was selected to represent Germany in the 1908 London Games, although he appears not to have competed in London (like Mallwitz, he also joined the Nazi Party, becoming an SS doctor and consultant to Himmler on matters relating to homosexuality) (www.olympedia.org). August Bier, who together with Mallwitz organised the first lectures in sports medicine at Berlin University in 1919, was an 'enthusiastic amateur' in 50 km running and also enjoyed several other sports including skating, sailing and swimming (Van Zundert, 2000). The physicians Ludwig Aschoff and Oskar de la Camp, who

DOI: 10.4324/9781003563921-7

played a key part in establishing what became the celebrated (and later, because of associated doping scandals, the infamous) sports medicine centre at Freiburg University, were also 'ambitious sportsmen' (Berg and König, 2002: 2). The physician Ernst Jokl, who was appointed in 1931 as director of the Institute of Sports Medicine at the University of Breslau, was an elite athlete who, three years earlier, had been selected as a reserve for Germany in the 400 metres hurdles at the 1928 Amsterdam Olympic Games (Carter, 2012: 69).

This symbiotic relationship between personal experience of and enthusiasm for modern sport and an interest in sports medicine was not, however, a characteristic of German sports medicine alone, for this personal, experiential element was a feature of sports medicine in other countries too. We noted in Chapter 3 that in England the limited qualified medical care that was available at sporting events was often provided on a voluntary basis by doctors who played, or had played, sport and who were enthusiastic supporters of what they saw as an exciting and pleasurable form of leisure activity. This passion for competitive sport was also a marked feature of the two most high-profile figures in the development of sports medicine in Britain, Adolphe Abrahams and Arthur (later Lord) Porritt, who were co founders of the British Association of Sport and Medicine and both of whom had an important influence not only on sports medicine in Britain but also worldwide (Carter, 2012: 72; Gerard, 1994: 77).

Adolphe Abrahams was a keen athlete and a member of a highly talented sporting family. At university he represented his Cambridge College and also won the Inter-Hospital Championships (Abrahams, 1968). Two of his younger brothers, Sidney and Harold, were elite athletes. Sidney competed in the 1912 Stockholm Olympics, while Harold won the gold medal in the 100 metres in the 1924 Paris Olympics, immortalised in the film, *Chariots of Fire*. Adolphe travelled with the UK athletics team at the 1908 and 1912 Olympics and later, and more formally, became an Honorary Medical Officer for the British Olympic Association from 1924 (Heggie, 2011: 62).

Arthur Porritt, like Abrahams, was a 'founding figure of sports medicine in the UK' (Gerard, 1994: 77) and 'As was the case with many of the early sports medicine practitioners, Porritt had a personal interest in sport' (Heggie, 2011: 102). He was in fact a highly talented and successful elite athlete, winning the bronze medal behind Harold Abrahams in the 100 metres race in the 1924 Olympic Games.

In France, the work of Viaud (2009a, 2009b) has emphasised the close relationship between the sporting activities of doctors and their practice of sports medicine. Many physicians combined a professional with a more personal interest in and passion for sport. Prominent examples include Marc Bellin du Côteau and Eugène Olivier. Du Côteau qualified as a doctor in 1910 and wrote several books on medical aspects of sport and physical education. He took a particular interest in the debate about 'athletes' heart' and was responsible for the physical conditioning of French athletes for the Olympic Games of 1920. He was himself also an elite athlete, having been the French national champion at 400 metres in 1904 and 1907 and he competed in the 1906 Intercalated Games in Athens (www.olympia.org/athletes/79601). Eugène Olivier graduated in medicine in 1911 and later became a professor of anatomy at the École Normale d'Éducation Physique before becoming director of the Regional Institute of Physical Education (IREP). As a medical student and a young doctor he had a very distinguished sporting career, representing France in fencing between 1905 and 1914 and winning gold and bronze medals at the 1908 London Olympics. René Guillet was another doctor who played an important part in the development of sports medicine in France. He was director of the Institut d'Éducation Physique et Sportive at Lyon and later played a central role in founding the Lyonnaise Society of Sports Medicine (Fischer and Cao, 2010). As a medical student, Guillet had been a talented athlete, winning the French university championships in 1936 in the high jump, long jump, shot put, discus and javelin. Pierre Dumas, who was appointed as senior physician of the Tour de France in 1952, was also a successful athlete, being the holder of a black belt in judo (Fotheringham, 2002: 157).

However, whereas in England and France the close symbiotic relationship between a personal passion for sport and an interest in sports medicine developed in a largely spontaneous and informal way, in Germany this relationship was institutionalised much more formally. Pfister (2011: 280; emphasis added) has noted that at the annual meetings of the DÄB, in addition to the conference proceedings, 'sporting contests were held ... in which young sports physicians *had* to take part ... sports physicians were expected to demonstrate not only their academic competence but also their practical knowledge based on personal experience'. The DÄB was also involved in drawing up regulations governing eligibility to work as a sports physician. The basic requirement was completion of a 12 day medical training course, but there was also a further requirement: that sports physicians should have personal sporting experience. To this end, they were required to take part in different types of sport and, in addition, they had to pass a test in various sports and, if they were younger than 32, they had to meet the requirements of the examination for the 'German sports badge' (Pfister, 2011: 282–283).

This close association between personal experience of and enthusiasm for sport and the practice of sports medicine – whether it was expressed spontaneously, as in England and France, or as a formal requirement, as in Germany – raises a number of interesting questions. Hoberman has noted that one of the arguments used to support the view that sports physicians should themselves be athletes or former athletes was that a familiarity with the lived experience of the athlete was a prerequisite for treating the athlete-client. In this regard, he cites the opinion of the Berlin physiologist, René du Bois-Reymond, who stated that 'Without wishing to offend the medical establishment, it should be acknowledged that the judgement of an untrained layman regarding sport and its excesses is worth more than that of an inexperienced physician' (cited in Hoberman, 1992: 240). Hoberman suggests that this statement may, perhaps, have been aimed at those physicians who were opposed to competitive sport, but it is nevertheless a truly astonishing statement, not least because it runs directly counter to the central argument which has been used by every occupational group seeking to establish professional status: that its claim to recognition as a profession is based, above all else, on the possession of a body of expert knowledge, gained as a result of a long and intensive period of professional education; it is of course precisely this claim to specialised knowledge which provides the essential basis for the differentiation between professionals and unqualified 'quacks'. As Freidson (1970: 5) has noted, the pre-eminence of the medical profession in the modern world is based largely on a claim to expert authority, that is to say, 'medicine's knowledge about illness and its treatment is considered to be authoritative and definitive'. But, quite remarkably, and in an attempt to justify the requirement that sports physicians should themselves be, or have been, active athletes, du Bois-Reymond more or less discounts the value of this body of specialised knowledge, suggesting that the medical knowledge of the doctor who has not played sport is of less value than the view of the layperson who has played sport. That he was prepared to discount medical knowledge in this way suggests how important the link between playing (or having played) sport and the practice of sports medicine was held to be.

There are other issues associated with the centrality of this close relationship between personal experience of and enthusiasm for sport and the practice of sports medicine. Perhaps the first point to note is that sports medicine is unique in this respect. Other medical specialities have never had either a formal requirement, as in sports medicine in Germany, or any informal expectation as part of the occupational culture, as in sports medicine in many other countries, that doctors will have had similar kinds of personal experiences as the patients they are treating. There has, for example, never been a requirement or an expectation that specialists in obstetrics must themselves have given birth, that an oncologist must personally have had cancer, or that psychiatrists must themselves have experienced mental health problems. How, then, can we account for this unique situation in sports medicine?

In this regard, it is important to note that members of every occupation – or at least every occupation whose members seek some form of public recognition or status – require some shared definition and understanding of their work and professional interests. This shared understanding has several important functions: it serves to differentiate members of the group from members of other, and perhaps competing, occupational groups; it serves as a basis for the organisation of professional activities such as professional associations and conferences; and it serves as a basis for the development of a sense of professional identity and community. In the case of other medical specialities, this shared definition and understanding of their work may be based upon a focus on particular parts of the body (e.g. cardiology, ophthalmology), or on particular types of diseases (oncology, infectious diseases, psychiatry), or on particular parts of the life-cycle in which the patient is held to be 'special' and therefore in need of particular forms of care (paediatrics, geriatric medicine).

None of these considerations could be readily applied to sports medicine. It did not focus on particular parts of the body. It did not focus on particular illnesses or injuries; indeed, as we noted earlier, there was no recognition at this time, by either the athletes or the attending doctors, that injuries resulting from sporting activities were sports-specific, or that they required any special forms of treatment. And it did not claim to treat a group of patients who could be considered 'special' in any way, for the view of the athletic body as the 'normal' body persisted well into the twentieth century with, at this time, no suggestion that the athlete was a 'special' patient who required special treatment, in the way in which children and elderly people were defined as 'special' in the developing specialist areas of paediatrics and geriatric medicine.

If sports physicians could not claim that there was anything special about the patient group which they treated, neither could they claim to offer any distinctive medical skills. As we noted earlier, Dr Walter Schnell, the president of the DÄB, had written in 1925 that the 'specific nature of the sports medical examination does not involve the development of a specialized method, but rather the application of established medical science of a specific area' (cited in Hoberman, 1992: 241). Nor could they even claim to offer a common set of medical skills in the way in which other groups of specialists, such as oncologists, or dermatologists, could lay claim to a specific shared body of knowledge and skills within their specialities. Pfister (2011: 279, 282) has pointed out that those doctors who were involved in sports medicine had 'diverse interests', adding that doctors 'in various branches of medicine from gynaecology and internal medicine to surgery contributed to the discussions on sports medicine'. This was certainly the case both in Germany and elsewhere.

Among the pioneers of sports medicine in Germany, August Bier was a distinguished surgeon who performed the first operation with spinal anaesthesia and who is noted particularly for his contribution to the development of modern anaesthesia (Van Zundert, 2000). Ludwig Aschoff was a pathologist and a professor of morbid anatomy (Rolleston, 1942). Rene du Bois-Reymond was a physiologist. Ernst Jokl was a specialist in internal medicine and neurology (Litsky, 1997). Walter Schnell had a varied career, working in the First World War as a medical officer in the German army and air force and afterwards working in the University Clinic in Frankfurt am Main and a Physiological Institute in Münster. He also developed expertise in aviation medicine and became a city medical officer in Halle. This diversity of medical interests also characterised sports medicine pioneers outside of Germany. In Britain, Adolphe Abrahams was a general physician with a particular interest in gastroenterology, while Arthur Porritt was a surgeon who became particularly concerned at the mutilation involved in radical mastectomy procedures for breast cancer and who developed a more conservative and aesthetic approach to breast surgery (Beasley, 2013).

Given the diverse range of medical interests of doctors who took an interest in sports medicine, it is clear that there was no body of medical knowledge or skills which they could call their own or which they held in common, other than their basic qualification in medicine which they shared with every other qualified doctor and which could not, therefore, serve to differentiate them as a distinct group within the profession. And, as we have seen, they could not, like their colleagues in other specialist areas, claim to have a clear and distinct patient group. It is within this context that we can begin to understand the central importance of the requirement, or at least the expectation, that sports physicians should be active or former athletes. With nothing to distinguish their practice in medical or scientific terms from the practice of other doctors, and with no distinct patient group which they could define as their own, it was their practice of and passion for sport – and perhaps little else – which served to differentiate them as a group, and to provide a tentative sense of collective identity within an emerging professional community. In this sense, their shared passion for sport was not a trivial, or unimportant, or marginal aspect of sports medicine; it was the 'social glue' which defined the group, gave it meaning and held it together. It was, in Durkheim's (1933: 79) term, the *conscience collective*, a system of collective beliefs and sentiments which served to foster their integration into this newly emerging professional group.

But this passion for sport did not function simply to integrate this diverse group of doctors into an incipient professional community; perhaps even more importantly, it also bound the physician-athlete and the patient-athlete together in a new and distinctive type of doctor-patient relationship, for within this relationship, doctor and patient were bound together not merely by the common medical aim, found in all doctor-patient relationships, of helping the patient to recover, but also by a strong, *extra-medical* consideration: a shared love of sport and, more particularly, a quest for sporting excellence which, as we will see in the following chapter, became increasingly important in the second half of the twentieth century.

There can be little doubt about the importance of the integrative function of a shared love of sport and personal sporting involvement for the group of early practitioners of sports medicine. This is not to suggest, of course, that those who stressed the importance of physicians being practically involved in sport did so because they were consciously aware of the consequences of their actions for the group as a whole. In this connection, we are not suggesting, for example, that the requirement that German physicians had to take part in sport at their annual conferences, or as part of their training for practice in sports medicine, was a deliberate, thought-out strategy which was designed to differentiate the group from other groups of practitioners, or to foster the development of a group occupational identity, though we should not perhaps rule out the possibility that there may have been some awareness of these consequences. However, as numerous sociologists have pointed out, people's actions often have important social consequences of which they are unaware (Durkheim, 1933; Merton, 1936, 1957; Elias, 1978a). But, at least for the moment, the question as to the degree to which the integrative functions of sporting participation for the group as a whole were, in Merton's (1957) terms, manifest (intended and recognised) or latent (unintended and unrecognised) functions is a question which we are not in a position to answer.

We have suggested above that the shared passion for sport was not an unimportant or trivial aspect of sports medicine. Neither was it a short lived, transitory feature which was characteristic merely of the early phases of the development of sports medicine but, on the contrary, it became an important part of the occupational culture of sports medicine and remains an important feature of sports medicine today. This has been a clear finding among research which has examined the motivations of contemporary medical practitioners for becoming involved in the practice of sports medicine; in this regard, the studies by Waddington, Roderick and Parker (1999) of club doctors in English professional football, and Malcolm's

(2006) study of club doctors in professional rugby in England are particularly revealing. These studies are reviewed in detail in the concluding chapter, where we examine in detail their significance for the doctor-patient relationship in sport.

In the meantime, we might note that a good deal of data from contemporary France also indicate a close relationship between a passion for sport/playing sport and the practice of sports medicine. In France many leading sports physicians were, in their younger days, outstanding athletes. Jean-François Toussant is professor of cardiology at the University of Paris, holds a consultancy in sports medicine at the Hotel Dieu hospital and is one of France's leading researchers in this area. In the 1980s he was an international volleyball player for France and was a member of the Asnières team which won the national championship in 1984. Charles Yannick Guezennec is a professor of physiology with an international reputation in sports medicine. From the mid-1960s through to the early 1980s, he was a member of the French national team in the modern pentathlon. Dr François Lhuissier, who has been physician to the French Triathlon Federation since 2009 and has also worked as a team doctor in professional football in France, is a former national junior duathlon champion and has represented France in the world duathlon championships. Gérard Dine was one of the founders of the Institut de Médecine du Sport de Troyes in 1983, and has worked with the French national rugby team and as an adviser to numerous international sports federations. He was also an elite rugby player, playing 8 times for New Caledonia in 1978-79 and winning a bronze medal with the New Caledonia team at the Pacific Games in 1979.

More systematic data from France on the relationship between sports physicians' personal participation in sport and their practice of sport medicine is provided by Viaud's (2009a) analysis of sports physicians in the Loire region in 2007-2008. Of 136 doctors who answered a question about whether they had played sport in the past, 124 (91.1%) indicated they had previously played sport, while 121 out of 144 (84%) indicated they were still playing sport at the time of the study. And a significant number had played sport at a relatively high level. Of the 102 who answered a question about the level at which they had played in the past, no fewer than 17 (16.6%) had played at the national/international level, 31 (30.3%) had played at the regional/interregional level, 18 (17.6%) had played at the district/departmental level, while 36 (35.2%) had played sport as a leisure activity (Viaud, 2009a: 26).

It is clear that, from the early development of sports medicine, the professional involvement of doctors with athletes has been inextricably intertwined with what Elias (1987b: 73) has called 'the intrusion of heteronomous evaluations', that is, values and interests from outside the social institutions of science – in this case, their passion for competitive sport as an activity which they have personally found exciting and enjoyable. In this regard, it might be said that, from the beginning, the involvement of medical practitioners in sports medicine has involved a particular, and unstable, balance between the autonomous values of science and the heteronomous values associated with participation in and love of sport, values which they shared with large numbers of sporting enthusiasts in the wider society. This particular admixture of scientific/medical and non-medical sporting values has been an important catalyst in the development of sports medicine, but it has also been a problematic aspect of the development of sports medicine, not least because it has required practitioners of sports medicine to 'buy into' two rather different codes of ethics: medical ethics and the 'sport ethic', which involve elements which may not be readily compatible. What has proved to be a problematic relationship between medical ethics and the sport ethic within the practice of sports medicine will be examined in more detail in the concluding chapter.

The physician-athlete, sport and public health

This involvement in and passion for competitive sport is also central to understanding another key aspect of the development of sports medicine. We noted in Chapter 2 that Heggie (2011: 12) noted that it 'could have been possible for sports medicine to be constructed as a version of public health or healthy living, but that is not … what happened in Britain'. It is suggested here that central to understanding why this did not happen in Britain is the fact that many of the doctors who took an interest in the developing area of sports medicine – and more particularly those who were at the forefront of this development – brought with them a strong personal prior commitment to the value of competitive sport as an exciting and pleasurable activity rather than a prior interest in public health and a commitment to exercise as the basis of public health programmes. In this regard, the British experience was not unique.

In Germany, as in Britain, sports medicine could have been constructed as a version of public health or healthy living but, as in Britain, this proved not to be the case. As we saw in the previous chapter, for much of the nineteenth century, the predominant form of physical culture in Germany was German gymnastics (*Turnen*), a system of pedagogic exercises which was embedded within a public health framework. However, as modern competitive sports became increasingly popular in Germany, so a major conflict developed between those who located exercise within a public health framework and the physician-athletes, led by the former Olympic athlete Arthur Mallwitz and supported by the German Olympic Association, who emphasised the significance of sports medicine not for public health but for high level competitive sport. By the late 1920s and early 1930s, as we have seen, the balance of power within the DÄB had shifted decisively in favour of the latter, with a shift away from a focus on public health and towards competitive elite sport and questions of performance and performance enhancement in elite competitive sport. In Germany, as in Britain, it was those who brought a prior personal involvement in, and commitment to, competitive sport, rather than those who brought a primary interest in public health, who defined the development of sports medicine.

References

Abrahams, H. (1968), The changing face of international sport, The memorial lecture to the late Sir Adolphe Abrahams, *Bulletin of the British Association of Sport Medicine*, 1 January 1968, 164–168. http://bjsm.bmj.com/ on 3/8/2020.

Beasley, W. (2013), Saints and sinners: Arthur Espie Porritt, *The Royal College of Surgeons of England Bulletin*, 274–275. https://doi.org/10.1308/147363513X13690603817265 (accessed 28 February 2022).
Berg, A. and König, D (2002), History of sports medicine in Germany with special reference to the University of Freiburg, *European Journal of Sport Science*, 2 (4), 1–7.
Carter, N. (2012), *Medicine, Sport and the Body: A Historical Perspective*, London, Bloomsbury.
Durkheim, E. (1933), *The Division of Labor in Society,* Glencoe, Free Press.
Elias, N. (1978a), *What Is Sociology?* London, Hutchinson.
Elias, N. (1987b), *Involvement and Detachment,* Oxford, Blackwell.
Fischer, L-P. and Cao, A. (2010), Le chirurgien René Guillet (1913–2002): son action dans le maquis de l'Ain et du Haut-Jura en 1944, *Histoire des Sciences Médicales*, 44 (1), 79–84.
Fotheringham, W. (2002), *Put Me Back on My Bike*, London, Yellow Jersey Press.
Freidson, E. (1970), *Profession of Medicine: A Study of the Sociology of Applied Knowledge*, New York, Dodd, Mead.
Gerard, D. F. (1994), Obituary: The Lord Porritt GCMG GCVO CBE Bt, *British Journal of Sports Medicine*, 28 (2), 77–78.
Heggie, V. (2011), *A History of British Sports Medicine*, Manchester, Manchester University Press.
Hoberman, J. (1992), The early development of sports medicine in Germany, in J. W. Berryman and R. J. Park (eds), *Sport and Exercise Science: Essays in the History of Sports Medicine*, Urbana and Chicago, University of Illinois Press, 233–282.
Litsky, F. (1997), Dr Ernst F. Jokl, a pioneer in sports medicine, dies at 90, *New York Times*, 21 December 1997.
Malcolm, D. (2006), Sports medicine: a very peculiar practice? Doctors and physiotherapists in elite English rugby union, in S. Loland, B. Skirstad and I. Waddington (eds), *Pain and Injury in Sport: Social and Ethical Analysis*, London, Routledge, 165–181.
Merton, R. K. (1936), The unintended consequences of purposive social action, *American Sociological Review*, 1 (6), 894–904.
Merton. R. K. (1957), *Social Theory and Social Structure*, New York, Free Press.
Pfister, G. (2011), 'Sports' medicine in Germany and its struggle for professional status, *Canadian Bulletin of Medical History*, 28 (2), 271–292.
Rolleston, J. D. (1942), Prof. Ludwig Aschoff, *Nature*, 150, 3 October, 338.
Van Zundert, A. (2000), August Bier 1861–1949, *Regional Anesthesia and Pain Medicine*, 25 (1), 26–33.
Viaud, B. (2009a), Médicines du sport, sports de médicins: quand les biographies sportives s'invitent dans le jeu des carrières professionelles, *Sciences Sociales et Sport*, 1 (2), 129–169.
Viaud, B. (2009b), *Panser les deux mondes. Médecines et sports, entre principes hippocratiques et performances*, PhD Dissertation, Université de Nantes.
Waddington, I., Roderick, M. and Parker, G. (1999), *Managing Injuries in Professional Football: A Study of the Roles of the Club Doctor and Physiotherapist*, Leicester, Centre for Research into Sport and Society, University of Leicester.

Part 2

The post-1945 period

Sports medicine comes of age

6 The medicalisation of sport and the establishment of sports medicine from the 1950s

We have seen in previous chapters that Germany led the world in many aspects of the development of sports medicine in the inter-war period. We have also seen that German physicians played a major role in the establishment of AIMS in 1928. But we have also noted that, at that time, even in Germany, doctors who treated athletes – not least the president of the newly formed association of sports physicians, Dr Walter Schnell – were adamant that there was no basis on which the medical care of athletes could become a distinct medical speciality, for the treatment of athletes was not seen as involving any special methods, but simply the application of general medical procedures. And we have also seen that if sports medicine did not involve any special medical procedures, neither did it involve – as did other established specialist areas of practice – either a focus on particular parts of the body, or on particular types of diseases, or on particular parts of the life-cycle in which the patient is held to be 'special'. Indeed, the very opposite was true, for medical practitioners who treated athletes did not claim that they treated a group of patients who were in any way 'special', for the view of the athletic body as 'normal' persisted well into the twentieth century, with no suggestion that the athlete was a 'special' patient who required special treatment in the way in which babies and elderly people were defined as 'special'. Despite the many developments in sports medicine in the inter-war period, there was no clear scientific rationale nor any occupational ideology to justify the establishment of sports medicine as a distinct branch of practice.

The development of sports medicine as a distinct area of medical practice was dependent on the articulation and acceptance of an occupational ideology which, firstly, defined what was unique to the practice of sports medicine – that is to say, what distinguished it from other areas of medical practice – and, secondly, justified increasing medical intervention in all aspects of the athletes' training and competition. The key process at the heart of this development was the medicalisation of sport, a process which not only changed the nature of sports medicine as a form of practice, but which also changed the structure of the relationship between sports physicians and their athlete-patients; indeed, the key process in the medicalisation of sport was the *transformation of athletes into patients*. The analysis of this process of the medicalisation of sport constitutes the central theme of this chapter.

Heiss has distinguished three stages in the development of sports medicine in Germany: (i) the application of general medical knowledge to the athlete

DOI: 10.4324/9781003563921-9

(1912–c.1925); (ii) the acquiring of a more systematic understanding of the effects of sport on the human body (c.1925–1955); and (iii) the development of sports medicine as a distinct branch of medical practice (from c. 1965) (Hoberman, 1992: 243). Heggie (2011: 74–75) has suggested that it is possible to identify broadly comparable periods in the development of sports medicine in Britain. In other words, one cannot speak of the emergence of sports medicine as a distinct branch of medical practice until the 1960s at the earliest.

This is not to say that there were no significant developments in sports medicine between the establishment of AIMS/FIMs and the 1960s. It is certainly the case that, in the 30 or so years after the establishment of FIMS, there were many developments in research physiology and in other aspects of knowledge and practice which may be considered as aspects of the first two phases of Heiss's three-part developmental schema. There were also significant improvements in the organisation and provision of medical care to elite athletes. For example, the 1932 Los Angeles Olympics were the first to set up an Olympic village, which included the most comprehensive medical services ever provided for athletes, while at the 1936 Berlin Olympics there was a hospital in the stadium, with medical care provided by no fewer than 176 physicians (Heggie, 2011: 75–76). There were also significant developments in the institutional structure of sports medicine in several countries. For example, new national sports medicine associations were established in the inter-war period (e.g. Italian Sports Medicine Association in 1929; Polish Sports Medicine Association in 1937) and in the early post-war years (e.g. Swedish Association of Sports Medicine and the British Association of Sport and Medicine, both established in 1952, and the American College of Sports Medicine, established in 1954) (Malcolm, 2017: 37).

But none of these developments provided – or indeed, could provide – an answer to the key question which must be addressed before any area of practice can be regarded as a distinct medical speciality: what is distinctive about that particular branch of medical practice? That is, how does the practice of sports medicine differ from other branches of medical practice? In order to answer this question we need to examine the medicalisation process, firstly in relation to the medicalisation of society in general and, secondly, specifically in relation to the medicalisation of sport.

The medicalisation of life

In a very influential essay in medical sociology, Irving Zola (1972) argued that in modern industrial societies medicine has become a major institution of social control. This process, he argued, was a largely insidious and often undramatic one which was associated with the 'medicalizing' of much of daily living, a process which involves 'making medicine and the labels "healthy" and "ill" *relevant* to an ever increasing part of human existence' (Zola, 1972: 487). Central to the medicalisation process has been an expansion of the number and range of human conditions which are held to constitute 'medical problems', a label which, once attached, is sufficient to justify medical intervention. Zola cited four such problems: ageing, drug addiction, alcoholism and pregnancy, the first and last of which were once regarded as normal processes and the middle two as human foibles and weaknesses. This has now changed and medical specialties have emerged to deal with these conditions, one consequence of which has been to expand very considerably the number of people deemed to be in need of medical services. A similar process has occurred as a result of the development of 'comprehensive' and psychosomatic medicine, both of which have considerably expanded the areas of life which are held to be relevant to the understanding, treatment and prevention of disease. The development of preventive medicine, in particular, has justified increasing medical intervention in an attempt to change people's lifestyles, whether in the areas of diet, sleep, work, sexual relationships, exercise, tobacco and alcohol consumption, or in the areas of safer driving or the fluoridation of water supplies.

Following Zola's classic statement, the theme of the medicalisation of life was taken up by a number of other writers. For example, Waitzkin and Waterman (1974: 86–89) analysed this process in terms of what they called 'medical imperialism'. However, perhaps the most famous thesis of this kind is that associated with Ivan Illich. Illich argued that the medicalisation of life involves a number of processes, including growing dependence on professionally provided care, growing dependence on drugs, medicalisation of the lifespan, medicalisation of prevention and medicalisation of the expectations of lay people. One of the consequences has been the creation of 'patient majorities' for, argued Illich (1975: 56), people 'who are free of therapy-oriented labels have become the exception'. Large numbers of people are now regarded as requiring routine medical attention, not because they have any definable pathology, but 'for the simple fact that they are unborn, newborn, infants, in their climacteric, or old' (Illich, 1975: 44). In other words, the expansion of that which is deemed to fall within the province of medicine has expanded to the point where, as de Swaan (1988: 243) has put it, 'there remain only patients and those not yet patients'.

Conrad (2005: 3) has pointed out that this early work on medicalisation drew attention to 'the creation (or construction) of new medical categories with the subsequent expansion of medical jurisdiction. Concepts such as moral entrepreneurs, professional dominance and claims-making were central to the analytical discourse'. Clarke et al. (2003: 161) have similarly noted that, in the decades after the Second World War, the 'growth of medicalisation – defined as the processes through which aspects of life previously outside the jurisdiction of medicine come to be construed as medical problems – is one of the most potent social transformations of the last half of the twentieth century' and they add that 'medicalization – the expansion of medical jurisdiction, authority, and practices into new realms – became widespread'. One of those new realms was sport.

The medicalisation of sport

Of central importance to the medicalisation of sport was a growing claim by sports physicians that – contrary to what had been held to be the case throughout most of the first half of the twentieth century – the athletic body was *not* a 'normal' body, that is to say, it was held to be different from the bodies of other, 'normal' people. This idea provided, for the first time, a clear rationale for the development of sports medicine as a distinct branch of practice, for the implication of this claim was that since the body of the athlete was not normal, but 'special', the athlete therefore required 'special' treatment. Although it has been suggested that one can identify the first signs of the development of this idea in the inter-war period (Heggie, 2011: 79–82), this idea was not articulated as a coherent occupational ideology until after the Second World War, and more particularly, until the 1960s. And under the umbrella of this new occupational ideology there took place the rapid development, particularly from the 1960s, of what is now recognised as sports medicine, an area of practice which was defined by two of the earliest and most prominent of British exponents (Williams and Sperryn, 1976: ix) as 'an integrated multidisciplinary field embracing the relevant areas of clinical medicine (sports traumatology, the medicine of sport and sports psychiatry) and the appropriate allied scientific disciplines (including physiology, psychology and biomechanics)'.

The key processes involved in the medicalisation of sport – and in particular the development of an ideology justifying increasing medical intervention – can be illustrated by reference to some of the early British textbooks in the area of sports medicine. This ideology is clearly expressed in one of the very first British texts in the field – J. G. P. Williams's *Sports Medicine,* which was published in 1962 – in which the author argues that the intensity and diversity of modern competitive sport have 'resulted in the emergence from the general mass of the population of a new type of person – the trained athlete'. Williams goes on to argue – some may feel that the case is overstated – that the trained athlete 'is as different physiologically and psychologically from "the man in the street" as is the chronic invalid'. This argument is, however, important in establishing a justification for medical intervention, for he goes on to suggest: 'Just as extreme youth and senility produce peculiar medical problems, so too does extreme physical fitness' (Williams, 1962: vii). One year after the publication of Williams's book, the same idea was expressed in a paper presented to a conference of the British Association of Sport and Medicine, held in Loughborough, in which it was argued that the 'trained athlete differs from the "average" member of the population as regards his physiology and responses to injury and illness as much as does a child or an older person' (cited in Heggie, 2011: 132). One can see here the early development of the idea, now widely accepted, that athletes require continual medical support not because they necessarily have any clearly defined pathology but, in this case, *simply because they are athletes*. This position was, in fact, spelt out quite unambiguously in the foreword to Williams's book by Sir Arthur (later Lord) Porritt who, as we noted earlier, had been a co-founder of the British Association of Sport and Medicine (BASM) and who was at that time the President of the Royal College of Surgeons of England and the Chairman of BASM. Porritt's position could hardly have constituted a clearer statement of what is involved in the medicalisation process, for he asserted quite simply that 'those who take part in sport and play games are essentially patients' (in Williams, 1962: v). Athletes thus became yet one more group to add to Illich's list of those – the unborn, newborn, infants and so on – who are held *by definition* to require routine medical supervision, irrespective of the presence or absence of any specific pathology.

It is important to note that the articulation of this occupational ideology not only radically extended the physicians' professional role and responsibilities in relation to athletes, but it also necessarily changed the nature of the relationship between physicians and their athlete-patients. For example, one consequence of the expansion of the physicians' role and their growing involvement with athletes (and also of the development from the 1960s of closely associated disciplines such as exercise physiology, biomechanics and sports psychology) was very quickly to make traditional methods of training for sporting events inadequate as a means of preparation for high-level competition. At the higher levels of sport the traditional image of the dedicated athlete training alone or with one or two chosen friends rapidly became outmoded. Instead, the modern successful athlete soon became surrounded by, and increasingly dependent upon, a whole group of specialist advisers, including specialists in sports medicine.

One result of these developments was that, from the 1960s, top-class athletes became more and more dependent on increasingly sophisticated systems of medical support in their efforts to run faster, to jump further or to compete more effectively in their chosen sport; by 1976, the President of the International Olympic Committee (IOC) Medical Commission was already able to observe that 'Modern top competition is unimaginable without doctors' (cited in Todd and Todd, 2001: 74). The former Amateur Athletics Association national coach, Ron Pickering, similarly noted in his foreword to Sperryn's *Sport and Medicine* (1983: vi) that few would deny that 'nowadays medical support is essential for the realization of the athlete's natural capacity for optimum performance'; indeed, at the highest levels of competition the quality of the medical support could make the difference between success and failure. Just how sophisticated those systems of medical backup had already become was illustrated by Pickering's admittedly tongue-in-cheek comparison between the limited amount of scientific knowledge which had been available to coaches at the start of his career as a coach in the early 1960s and the vast amount of knowledge which had subsequently been gained from experiments on athletes 'who have given blood, sweat, urine, muscle biopsies and personality inventories, have often been immersed in tanks, and photographed naked in three dimensions at altitude'.

It is important to note that this growing dependence of athletes on practitioners of sports medicine quickly went beyond the treatment of sports injuries for, as another early British text pointed out, as

> practice for the competitive event takes place … the sportsman [sic] seeks systematic methods of preparation. He examines such technical and scientific information as is available about the way his body performs its athletic function and turns to the doctor as physiologist.
>
> (Williams and Sperryn, 1976: 1)

In other words, the role of the sports physician was extended beyond simply treating injuries; performance enhancement became formally recognised as a key part of the role of the sports physician. That the role of sports physicians in enhancing performance is now clearly institutionalised as part of the practice of sports medicine is indicated by the British Medical Association's definition of sports medicine, which explicitly recognises that it is concerned not just with the 'prevention, diagnosis, and treatment of exercise related illnesses and injuries' but also with the 'maximization of performance' (BMA, 1996: 4). Similarly FIMS, on its website, says that it 'aims primarily to promote the study and development of sports medicine throughout the world … and *to assist athletes in achieving optimal performance* by maximising their genetic potential, health, nutrition and (access to) high-quality care and training' (FIMS, 2023: emphasis added). As Safai (2007: 326) has noted in her study of the development of sports medicine in Canada, sport medicine became 'a tool to be used in the enhancement of athletes' performance in training and competition'.

It would, however, be quite wrong to suggest that athletes are simply unwilling 'victims' of medical imperialism for, as de Swaan (1988: 246) has noted, professionals – in this instance, doctors – 'do not simply force themselves upon innocent and unknowing clients'. In the case of sport, a number of developments, particularly in the post-1945 period, have increasingly led athletes to embrace the help of anyone who can hold out the promise of improving their level of performance. The most important of these developments are probably those which have been associated with the politicisation of sport, particularly at the international level, and those which have been associated with massive increases in the rewards – particularly, but not exclusively, the material rewards – associated with sporting success. Both these processes, it is suggested, have had the consequence of increasing the competitiveness of sport, and one aspect of this increasing competitiveness has been the downgrading, in relative terms, of the traditional value associated with taking part while greatly increasing the value attached to winning. The increasing competitiveness of modern sport has had a significant impact on both athletes and sports physicians, and on the relationship between them, and for this reason it is important to analyse briefly some key aspects of this process.

The politicisation of sport

The relationship between politics and sport is of course not exclusively a post-Second World War phenomenon – note, for example, the 'Nazi Olympics' of 1936 (Mandell, 1987). However, there can be little doubt that sport has become increasingly politicised in the period since 1945. Of particular significance in this regard was the development of communist regimes in many parts of Eastern Europe and, associated with this, the emergence of the Cold War and of superpower rivalry. Within this context, international sporting competition took on a significance going far beyond the bounds of sport itself, for sport – at least within the context of East-West relations – became to some extent an extension of the political, military and economic competition which characterised relationships between the superpowers and their associated blocs.

The Helsinki Olympics of 1952 were the first Olympics at which Western athletes competed against athletes from the Soviet Union. With this development, the Olympics 'took on a new political dimension ... one that was destined to grow increasingly important in the decades to follow' (Guttmann, 1992: 97). The athletes were clearly aware of this new dimension. Guttmann suggests that the American winner of the decathlon in those Olympics, Bob Mathias, spoke for many when he wrote:

> There were many more pressures on American athletes because of the Russians ... They were in a sense the real enemy. You just loved to beat 'em. You just had to beat 'em ... This feeling was strong down through the entire team.

The Soviet athletes, for their part, were housed not in the Olympic Village, where they might have interacted with fellow athletes from the rest of the world, but in their own isolated quarters near the Soviet naval base at Porkkala, while the Soviet officials 'seemed to care only for the gold medals needed to certify the superiority of "new socialist man"' (Guttmann, 1992: 97). Meanwhile, newspapers 'concentrated on the "battle of the giants" and published daily statistics on the number of unofficial points earned by the United States and the Soviet Union' (Guttmann, 1992: 98).

Comparisons of the number of Olympic medals won by the United States and the Soviet Union thus came to be very important, for the winning of medals came to be seen as a symbol not only of national pride but also of the superiority of one political system over another. This East-West competition was further intensified following the admission of separate teams from West Germany and East Germany from the 1968 Olympics (Hill, 1992: 39); in East Germany the outstanding Olympic performances of their 'diplomats in tracksuits' were seen as crucial in breaking the international isolation of East Germany (Dennis, 2015: 170). As many governments came to see international sporting success as an important propaganda weapon in the East-West struggle, those athletes who emerged as winners came increasingly to be treated as national heroes with rewards – sometimes provided by national governments – to match. And as we will see in the next chapter (in the case studies of East Germany, and of the role of Dr Ziegler in the development of the anabolic steroid Dianabol for the use of American athletes) and in Chapter 8 (in the case study of sports medicine in France) the close entanglement of national prestige, international politics and sport had a significant impact not only on elite athletes but also on the development of sports medicine and on the practice of sports physicians.

Sport and commercialisation

The increase in the competitiveness of international sport has also been associated with the growing commercialisation of sport, particularly since the 1970s, and particularly in the West. Central to the commercialisation of sport have been two processes: the development of sports sponsorship and the increasing global audience, *via* television, for both live and recorded sport. From the 1970s, the growth in these two areas was so rapid that, by 2001–2004, corporate sponsorship and the sale of television rights together already accounted for 87 per cent of the income of the Olympic Movement. The growth of sports sponsorship was quite spectacular in the last decades of the twentieth century; Gratton and Taylor noted that while sports sponsorship 'hardly existed as an economic activity before 1970 in Britain' by the end of the century, it was estimated to be worth £350 million' (Gratton and Taylor, 2000: 163). The value of sports sponsorship has continued to grow rapidly in the first two decades of the twenty-first century; in 2012 the global sports sponsorship market was worth $51.1 billion (Donlan, 2014), increasing to $66 billion in 2022 (Gough, 2024) with, perhaps not surprisingly, the United States having the highest share of sports sponsorship.

The commercialisation of sport has, particularly from the 1970s, underpinned a massive increase in the non-honorific rewards – and in particular the financial rewards – associated with Olympic success. Although this development appears to be a fairly general one within Western societies, the financial rewards associated with Olympic success are probably greatest in the United States. By 1990, Robert Voy, a former chief medical officer to the US Olympic team, was able to point to the huge financial rewards which had by then become available in the United States to Olympic gold medal winners, who were able not only to demand very high appearance fees for competing in major meetings but, much more importantly, could also earn huge incomes from sponsorship, from television commercials and from product endorsement. However, Voy went on to point out that such fabulous rewards were available only to those who come first for, as he put it, 'second place doesn't count' (Voy, 'On the Line', 1990).

In their history of sports in America since 1945 – significantly entitled *Winning is the Only Thing* – Roberts and Olsen summarise the impact of the political and economic processes outlined above on the growing competitiveness and seriousness of sport. They write:

> There was a time in United States history, back in the pre-World War II era, when sports knew its place in American culture. It was a pastime, diversion, leisure, recreation, play – fun. In sports people found relief from the real things of the world and their own lives – wars, unemployment, social conflict, politics, religion, work, prices, and family. But after World War II, sports assumed an extraordinary significance in people's lives; games became not only a reflection of the changes occurring in the United States but a lens through which tens of millions Americans interpreted the significance of their country, their communities, their families, and themselves. Americans came to take sports very seriously, and they watched and played for the highest economic, politic, and personal stakes.
>
> (Roberts and Olsen, 1989: xi–xii)

Leaving aside a hint of romanticism – and the rather strange implied suggestion that somehow sport before 1945 was not one of the 'real things' of the world – Roberts and Olsen do nevertheless highlight a very important change in the structure of sport in the post-1945 period. Sport is now more competitive and more serious than it used to be. A greater stress is laid upon the importance of winning. And sport is played for higher – sometimes much higher – stakes, whether these be economic, political or personal.

It is important to note that these two key processes – the medicalisation of sport and the increasing seriousness and competitiveness of sport – provide the essential context for understanding what almost all academics who have studied doping, as well as anti-doping practitioners who have worked in this area, agree has been a very substantial increase in the use of performance-enhancing drugs by athletes from the 1960s (Donohoe and Johnson, 1986; Lüschen, 2000; Verroken, 2005; Donati, 2004; Yesalis and Bahrke, 2005; Waddington and Smith, 2009; Paoli and Donati, 2014, Paoli, 2019). In order to understand this argument more fully, it may be useful to revisit what might be called the sport/medicine axis.

The sport/medicine axis

At this stage it might be useful to summarise briefly the argument in this chapter thus far. We have suggested that the period since 1945, and in particular the period from the 1960s, was particularly significant in the development of both sport and sports medicine, and of the relationship between them, as a result of two processes. The first of these relates to the medicalisation of sport, while the second relates to the increasing competitiveness of sport and to a growing emphasis on the importance of winning. It is suggested that the first of these processes – the medicalisation of sport – has meant that medical practitioners have become increasingly prepared to make their professional knowledge and skills available to athletes, while the second process – the increasing competitiveness of modern sport – has meant that athletes have become increasingly eager to seek the help of scientists who could improve the level of their performance. The conjuncture of these two processes, it is suggested, has been associated with two closely related developments. One of these developments has involved the increasing application of the growing knowledge within disciplines such as exercise physiology and biomechanics in the search for enhanced performance; the other development has involved the increasing use by athletes of an increasing variety of pharmacological products, both licit and illicit, to improve their performance. And the evidence is unambiguously clear: practitioners of sports medicine have been centrally involved not only in the first, but also in the second, of these developments.

The relationship between processes of medicalisation and drug use has been noted by Houlihan (2002: 30) who stressed that the use of performance-enhancing drugs:

> needs to be seen in the context of an increasingly pill-dependent society. It is unrealistic to expect athletes to insulate themselves from a culture which expects pharmacists and doctors to be able to supply medicines for all their ills whether physical or psychological.

Houlihan adds that 'it is also unrealistic to ignore the importance of legitimate drugs in the intensely scientific training regimes of most, if not all, elite athletes'. In this regard, it is important to note that the development of sports medicine has been associated with the development of a culture which encourages the treatment not just of injured athletes, but also of healthy athletes, with drugs. As Houlihan has noted:

> Even if the 'drugs' are simply those which are legally available … such as vitamins and food supplements, the athlete is already developing the expectations and patterns of behaviour that might initially parallel illegal drug use, but which are to most athletes part of a common culture.
>
> (Houlihan, 2002: 100–101)

This point was nicely illustrated by Dr Robert Voy when he recorded the daily intake of legal drugs of a national American track star: vitamin E, 160 mg; B-complex capsules, four times per day; vitamin C, 2000 mg; vitamin B6, 150 mg; calcium tablets, four times per day; magnesium tablets, twice a day; zinc tablets, three times a day; royal jelly capsules; garlic tablets; cayenne tablets; eight aminos; Gamma-Oryzanol; Mega Vit Pack; super-charge herbs; Dibencozide; glandular tissue complex; natural steroid complex; Inosine; Orchid testicle extract; Pyridium; Ampicillin; and hair rejuvenation formula with Biotin (Voy, 1991: 99).

It should be noted that since the analysis offered here stresses the conjuncture of two processes, one within the world of medicine and the other within the world of sport, it follows that the increasing use of drugs in sport since the 1960s *cannot be explained simply by reference to the changing patterns of behaviour amongst athletes*. Rather, it is argued that the increasing use of illicit drugs has been associated with the emergence, in both the world of sport and the world of medicine, of those who may be described as innovators or entrepreneurs. Within the world of sport, it is perhaps not surprising that, given the increased emphasis which has come to be placed on winning, an increasing number of athletes have been prepared to innovate by making illicit use of the fruits of medical and pharmacological research. Equally, however, it is a clear implication of the above analysis that there are doctors – and again their number has almost certainly increased substantially since the 1960s – who may be regarded as medical 'entrepreneurs' in the sense that they are prepared to stretch the boundaries of 'sports medicine' to include the prescribing of drugs with the specific intention of improving athletic performance. This point is of some importance for it suggests that the use of drugs in sport has been associated with the development of a network of co-operative relationships between innovators or entrepreneurs from the two increasingly closely related fields of sport and medicine. What is the evidence for this?

Doctors as providers of 'chemical assistance'

There is a good deal of direct evidence relating to the involvement of doctors in the use of drugs in elite sport, particularly since the 1960s. In this regard, the Dubin Commission of Inquiry, established by the Canadian Government following Ben Johnson's infamous positive test at the 1988 Seoul Olympics, was a watershed, for it provided detailed evidence of the networks of relationships of those, including medical practitioners, involved in drug use in Canada and the United States. Even before the Dubin Commission, however, there was already growing evidence of the involvement of physicians in the use of drugs in sport. One early example was the work of Dr John Ziegler who, in the 1950s, was involved in developing anabolic steroids for the use of American weightlifters. We also know that physicians were involved in blood doping the United States cycling team at the 1984 Los Angeles Olympics, while evidence of the systematic involvement of doctors in doping in Eastern Europe from the 1970s was already beginning to emerge, often as a result of the defection of sportspeople to the West, in the 1980s. These three instances shed a good deal of light on the changing relationship between elite-level athletes and practitioners of sports medicine, and they provide the basis for three detailed case studies in the next chapter.

Since the 1970s there have been many other well-documented examples of the involvement of physicians in the use of drugs in sport. Within Britain, *The Times* newspaper in 1987 published a three-part investigation into drug use in British sport, in which it claimed that 'there is little doubt' that many British international athletes used drugs, a conclusion which, it claimed, was confirmed by 'athletes with whom we spoke, by coaches who advise them and by doctors who both monitor and supply them' (16 December 1987). Following these revelations in *The Times*, the Amateur Athletics Association established a committee of enquiry chaired by Peter Coni, a barrister and former rower. In its report the Coni Enquiry confirmed that there was indeed widespread drug use in at least some sports within Britain and that this had increased from the late 1950s and 1960s. Of particular relevance within the present context is that the Coni Enquiry also accepted another key claim of *The Times* articles: that there were doctors in Britain who were involved in 'monitoring athletes on a regular basis in circumstances which can only be construed as checking the effect upon those athletes of the drugs they have been taking to aid their performances' (Coni, Kelland and Davies, 1988: para. B20). The report concluded in relation to the involvement of doctors that:

> We have evidence of a few doctors prepared to prescribe banned drugs to athletes … Medical support arises more often, though, on the basis of the doctor who says that, whilst he would never advocate the taking of drugs for the sake of athletic achievement, it is his responsibility if an athlete has made that decision for himself to monitor the athlete's health to ensure so far as the doctor can that he does so without physical harm. Since availability of banned drugs presents few problems, the end result from the standpoint of drug use by athletes – that medical advice is available for those who care to look for it – is of course the same, whether the doctor is prescribing, or simply monitoring the effects.
>
> (para. B21)

As we will see in the case study of sports medicine in France in later chapters, the argument that monitoring by doctors of drug use by athletes could reduce the health risks to athletes was an argument that was regularly used by sports physicians in France in the 1960s and 1970s to justify their involvement in doping.

Several years after the Coni Enquiry, *The Times* revealed that Dr Jimmy Ledingham, who was a doctor to the British Olympic men's team between 1979 and 1987, had provided steroids to British athletes, monitored the effects of the drugs on them and given them advice on how to avoid testing positive (29 October 1995).

The Dubin Commission, which took evidence under oath, provided perhaps the clearest and most detailed picture of the network of relationships between doctors, athletes and coaches in relation to drug use. Angela Issakenko, who was the first of the athletes coached by Charlie Francis to use anabolic steroids, testified to the Commission that she obtained her first prescription for Dianabol from Dr Gunther Koch, a physician practising in Toronto, in 1979. In 1983, she went on a different drug programme following a visit to Dr Robert Kerr in San Gabriel, California, while from the autumn of 1983 until 1988, her drug programme was supervised by Dr Jamie Astaphan, who also supervised the drug programme of Ben Johnson (Dubin, 1990: 244–246).

In his evidence to the Dubin Commission, Dr Astaphan indicated that a number of Canada's leading track and field athletes had consulted him, and that he had provided them with advice and assistance in regard to anabolic steroids and other performance-enhancing drugs. Astaphan testified that he had also been consulted by athletes from the United States and from many countries in Europe and Africa. They included athletes in a number of sports; in addition to advising athletes in track and field, Astaphan also supervised drug programmes for football players, weightlifters, powerlifters and bodybuilders (Dubin, 1990: 251).

Elsewhere in its report, the Dubin Commission noted that the 'names of physicians willing to prescribe anabolic steroids and other performance-enhancing drugs circulate widely in gyms' and that such physicians 'may develop practices with a focus on athletes and performance-enhancing drugs'. One such practitioner named in the report was Dr Ara Artinian, a Toronto-based practitioner who had been prescribing and administering anabolic steroids to athletes regularly for several years. That Artinian was prescribing for a substantial number of athletes is suggested by the fact that, between 1981 and 1988, he purchased anabolic steroids worth $215,101 from various pharmaceutical companies. He administered injections and provided pills to athletes in return for cash payments rather than providing a prescription to fill at a pharmacy. Artininian worked mainly with football players and bodybuilders rather than athletes in Olympic sports (Dubin, 1990: 356).

The Commission also took evidence from Bruce Pinnie, a former shot-putter who at the time of the inquiry was a throwing coach, and who testified that he had obtained anabolic steroids for performance-enhancement purposes from his doctor as early as 1972. Pinnie indicated that there were, even at that early date, several doctors in Winnipeg who were well known for their willingness to supply steroids

(Dubin, 1990: 356–357). In relation to the situation in Canada the Dubin report noted that:

> The Commission also heard evidence from many other athletes that they received anabolic steroids directly from physicians. Clearly, there are physicians in most major centers across the country who have at one time or another been involved in prescribing anabolic steroids and other performance-enhancing drugs to athletes.
>
> (Dubin, 1990: 357)

Dubin also pointed out that the situation in the United States appeared to be similar. The shot-putter and discus thrower, Peter Dajia, described visiting a doctor's office in Fort Worth, Texas, and obtaining a prescription for anabolic steroids simply by indicating what he wanted. Particularly revealing was the evidence of Dr Robert Kerr, a California sports physician, who estimated that there were at least seventy physicians in the Los Angeles area alone who prescribed anabolic steroids to athletes. Kerr, who was the author of *The Practical Use of Anabolic Steroids with Athletes* and who was often referred to as the 'steroid guru', had an extensive practice principally involving US athletes, though he indicated that he had also prescribed anabolic steroids for athletes from Canada, South America, Australia and the Far East (Dubin, 1990: 357). In his evidence, Kerr also testified that he had prescribed anabolic steroids to approximately twenty medallists at the 1984 Olympic Games (Armstrong, 1991: 61).

Dubin also noted that in Australia, a senate Committee investigating the use of drugs in sport had estimated that 15,000 users obtained anabolic steroids through physicians. Forty-one per cent of a group of Australian bodybuilders who were surveyed indicated that physicians were their source of supply. One medical witness who gave evidence to Dubin stated that in Sydney there were between 10 and 20 doctors who prescribed anabolic steroids, and that he himself would see up to 200 'patients' a year for this purpose. Another medical witness testified that he was prescribing anabolic steroids for 50 male bodybuilders, 1 female weightlifter and 3 other athletes (Dubin, 1990: 357).

Ben Johnson's positive drug test at the Seoul Olympics was, in a number of respects, a watershed in the history of drug use in sport. The event generated huge media coverage – Johnson was, after all, the then reigning world champion, world record holder and 'winner' of the Olympic final and, as such, he had an undisputed claim to be 'the fastest man on earth' – and it raised public awareness of the use of drugs in elite sport to a level which was almost certainly unprecedented. The establishment of the Commission of Inquiry under Mr Justice Dubin, which followed Johnson's disqualification, also marked a watershed in some respects, for it provided more systematic, more reliable and more detailed information about the network of relationships among those involved in drug use – and particularly the involvement of doctors – than had ever been available before.

However, the revelations contained in the Dubin report did little, if anything, to disrupt what was by then a well-established pattern of relationships between doctors and drug-using athletes. Seven years after Dubin reported, the *British Journal of Sports Medicine* published a study of drug use among 2000 amateur athletes in France which found that doctors were by far the most common source of drugs; of the 186 athletes who admitted using banned substances, no fewer than 61 per cent reported that they had obtained their drugs from a doctor compared with just 20 per cent who obtained them on the black market. And since the drugs were prescribed within the framework of the French national health insurance scheme, the cost of the drugs was reimbursed by social security! (Laure, 1997).

The year after Laure's study was published, the drugs scandal in the 1998 Tour de France made it unambiguously clear that, once again, physicians – this time in the form of team doctors – were heavily implicated in the organisation of drug use. Since this constitutes a detailed case study in Chapter 10, we will not examine the 1998 Tour de France in detail here, but for the moment we simply wish to note the central involvement of team doctors. The team at the heart of the scandal was Festina, whose *soigneur* (masseur) was arrested *en route* to the start of the Tour when French police found 250 batches of anabolic steroids and 400 ampoules of EPO in his car. It quickly emerged that there was, within the Festina team, a systematic programme of drug use by team members which was organised by the team director, Bruno Roussel, and the team doctor, Eric Rijkaert; the objective of this system was, according to Roussel, 'to improve performances under strict medical control in order to avoid the unauthorised personal supply to cyclists causing grave attacks to their health' (*Sunday Telegraph*, 19 July 1998). As we have noted earlier, Roussel's claim that medical control of the doping process reduced harm to the athletes' health had long been a refrain by practitioners of sports medicine in France and elsewhere. Both Roussel and Rijkaert were charged by French police under the 1989 Anti-Drug Act, which prohibits the administration of doping substances or techniques. Three days later, the Dutch TVM team withdrew from the Tour following more drug use revelations and the TVM team doctor, Andrei Mikhailov, was also charged under French anti-doping laws after admitting supplying more than 100 doses of EPO which had been found in a TVM team vehicle. And before the Tour ended, another team doctor, Nicholas Torralbos of the ONCE team, which included the world-ranked number one cyclist, Laurent Jalabert, was also charged under the 1989 Act with supplying banned drugs (Waddington, 2000: 156–159).

Two years before the notorious 1998 Tour de France, two French professional cyclists, Phillippe Gaumont and Laurent Desbiens, tested positive for the steroid nandrolone, and it was subsequently revealed that the drug had been supplied by their team doctor, Patrick Nedelec, who had previously worked for both the French national cycling federation and also for the international governing body of cycling, the Union Cycliste Internationale, which is the body responsible for drug testing within cycling! (*Cycling Weekly*, 29 June 1996). The 1998 Tour de France indicated very clearly that this practice was not unique to the team for which Gaumont and Desbiens raced, but that it was a common practice among professional teams on the European continent.

There is, too, abundant evidence of medical involvement in drug use in Italian sport. In 2004, in an investigation of allegations of doping at the leading Italian football club, Juventus, a police raid ordered by the Turin public attorney revealed that the club held no fewer than 281 different pharmacological products, including some banned substances (*The Times*, 1 December 2004); at the subsequent trial, one witness suggested that 'either the players were always sick or they took drugs without justification ... to enhance performance' (*Sports Illustrated,* 7 December 2005). The club's managing director, Antonio Giraudo, and the club doctor, Riccardo Agricola, were charged with supplying pharmacological products to several players between 1994 and 1998, a period during which Juventus won three Italian titles and the European Cup. At the trial evidence was presented that some players, and perhaps as many as 20, had been involved in the 'chronic use' of erythropoietin, commonly called EPO. The club doctor was convicted under Italian law of supplying banned drugs to Juventus players and was given a 22-month suspended jail sentence, banned from practising medicine for 22 months and fined 2000 Euros (*Independent*, 1 December 2004; *Independent on Sunday,* 27 March, 2005).

The leading medical figure in doping in Italy since the 1970s has unquestionably been Dr Francesco Conconi, Professor of biochemistry at the University of Ferrara. In the late 1970s, Conconi started providing a variety of doping products to Italian elite athletes in many sports with, it might be noted, the tacit support of CONI, the Italian Olympic Committee (Paoli, 2019: 83). Many details of the involvement of Conconi in doping were first revealed by the leading athletics coach and anti-doping campaigner, Alessandro Donati (Donati, 2004, 2006). Donati has recorded that in 1981, shortly after he became a national athletics coach, he was approached by Dr Conconi, who indicated that the Italian Athletics Federation had asked him to advise Donati about a project on which he was working. Conconi was one of the leading researchers in the area of blood doping and, like his colleagues in sports medicine in other countries, he was seeking to refine this technique, which involved giving athletes transfusions of their own blood a few days before a major event as a means of boosting the red blood cells and thereby increasing the amount of oxygen reaching the muscles. Donati and the athletes he was coaching considered this technique unethical and refused to participate in Conconi's work. However, Conconi continued to refine the technique, which he used in preparing the Italian cyclist Francesco Moser for his successful attempt in 1983 to break the world hour record which had been set 11 years earlier by Eddy Merckx.

Donati also records that, at about the same time, a physician and former decathlete, Daniele Faraggiana, had been instructed by the Italian Athletics Federation and the Weightlifting Federation to 'treat' the athletes of their respective national teams, mostly with anabolic steroids and testosterone. Donati obtained documents which not only revealed the names of the athletes involved and the drugs which were used, but also recorded that Faraggiana had supplied Conconi with banned substances. But perhaps most striking was the fact that the Anti-Doping Laboratory in Rome, which had been duly accredited by the IOC, 'was being used for a totally different purpose: to establish how long it would take for traces of these drugs to disappear from the athletes' urine samples' (Donati, 2004: 47).

Conconi continued to work with elite athletes throughout the 1990s, and was a central figure in developing the use of EPO for athletes. After many years campaigning by Donati, the Italian police in 1997 began a criminal investigation into Conconi's activities. The police seized files, revealing results of numerous blood tests on athletes in various sports, from Conconi's laboratory. Conconi was eventually charged in 2002 with drug-related offences in relation to 33 elite athletes, many of them cyclists, including the Irish cyclist Stephen Roche who in 1987 won both major tours – the Tour de France and the Giro d'Italia – and also the World Road Race Championship. Conconi's collaborator, Dr Giovanni Grazzi, a former physician to the Carrera cycling team, for whom Roche had ridden, was also charged with having administered doping substances. Following several delays associated with technical legal matters, the date for Conconi's trial was eventually set for October 2003 but the slowness of the Italian legal process meant that the case never came to court because the offences were covered by the Statute of Limitations; the charges and the written evidence related to actions which had taken place prior to August 1995 and they were therefore outside the period of limitation in Italian law. However, the judge, Judge Franca Oliver, issued what has been described as a 'damning verdict' on Conconi and his associates, of whom she said: 'It's clear that they knew all about the riders taking EPO and for years continuously supported and encouraged them with tests and analysis to optimise their results in races'. She added that they 'kept detailed computer records of athletes' blood values so they could optimise and keep control of the doping product erythropoietin' (*Cycle Sport*, May 2004). Donati writes: 'Although seven years of investigation and prosecution … had confirmed the responsibilities of … Prof. Conconi and his associates, they all managed to avoid being convicted thanks to the Statute of Limitations' (Donati, 2004: 55).

It is important to note that Conconi was not a fringe practitioner of sports medicine but, on the contrary, one who worked at the very heart of the sports medicine establishment; he was a member of the Medical Committee of the International Olympic Committee (IOC) and the President of the Medical Commission of the Union Cycliste Internationale (UCI). His research had also been funded for 20 years by the Italian Olympic Committee and he had also received large amounts of funding from the IOC, supposedly to develop a test for erythropoietin (EPO) which he never delivered. As Donati has noted, it would have been extremely embarrassing for the Italian sporting authorities, for the IOC and for the governing body of cycling, the UCI, if the trial had gone ahead, for Conconi had for many years been a pillar of the sports medicine establishment not just in Italy but also internationally.

Dr Michelle Ferrari was the most famous of Conconi's pupils and from the late 1990s he worked with many of the world's leading cyclists (as we shall see in Chapter 10, one of his 'patients' was Lance Armstrong). Like Conconi, Ferrari eventually became the subject of a criminal investigation which resulted in 2004 in a conviction for sporting fraud and the illegal exercise of the pharmaceutical profession. Ferrari was given a one-year suspended sentence and a fine of 900 euros and was banned from practising as a sports doctor in cycling by Italy's cycling Federation (*Sunday Times*, 3 October 2004). However, Ferrari ignored the ban and later worked with Lance Armstrong, where he was described by Armstrong's teammate Tyler Hamilton as 'our doctor, our god' (Hamilton and Coyle, 2012: 102). After the exposure of doping in Armstrong's team, and his central role in that, Ferrari accepted the charges and received a lifetime ban. Again, it is important to note that Ferrari, like Conconi, was not a marginal figure within sports medicine; not only was he working with the world's leading cyclist – Armstrong was the only cyclist to win the Tour de France seven times, though his victories were, of course, all subsequently annulled – but he was, in the words of the judge who sentenced him in 2004, one of 'the best sports physicians … trained at a centre of excellence funded by CONI' (Paoli and Donati, 2014: 72).

Dr Carlo Santuccione, who was a former assistant of Conconi and who was allegedly known as *Ali the Chemist*, was suspended from acting as a sports physician from 1995 to 2000 by CONI for a doping offence. Following this, from 2004 he was the central focus of a major police investigation into the large-scale prescription and sale of performance-enhancing drugs to at least 146 athletes in 29 Italian provinces; this investigation led to the seizure of very large quantities of doping products, totalling 38,059 doses of drugs and blood-doping equipment. Santuccione was suspected of coordinating the whole network of suppliers of performance-enhancing drugs and of connecting the athletes with their suppliers. In 2007 he was given a lifetime ban by CONI from all involvement in sport as a result of these charges (Paoli and Donati. 2014: 70).

Finally, from among many other examples of medical involvement which could be cited, reference should be made to the extensive blood doping network which was uncovered by the Spanish police in 2006. In 2004, Jesus Manzano, a former professional cyclist with the Spanish-based Kelme team spoke out about the use of drugs within his team and this led to a police investigation which centred on the Madrid clinic of Dr Eufemiano Fuentes, who worked with Jose Luis Merino Batres, the chief of haematology at a Madrid hospital. The police investigation, codenamed *Operación Puerto*, raided Fuentes' premises and found hundreds of packets of blood taken from athletes, each with a codename (which police were unable to decipher) to protect the identity of Fuentes' clients. The police operation revealed that Dr Fuentes had been involved in blood doping perhaps as many as 200 elite athletes, including many of the world's leading cyclists. Dr Fuentes was charged, not under anti-doping law – Spain had no anti-doping laws at that time – but under Spanish public health law. In the court case, Dr Fuentes admitted that he had been involved in doping athletes and offered to reveal the names of all his clients in elite sport but was told he was not legally obliged to do so. He was convicted and given a one-year suspended prison sentence but in 2016 the original verdict against Fuentes was overruled.

Conclusion

In this chapter we have argued that in the post-1945 period, but particularly in the period from the 1960s, the conjuncture of two processes – one within the world of medicine and the other within the world of sport – have brought sports physicians and athletes increasingly closely together in the search for enhanced performances. And we have set out a substantial body of evidence which, we suggest, indicates that the increased involvement of sports physicians in the search for enhanced sporting performance has involved significant numbers of doctors in the development and use of performance-enhancing drugs by athletes from the 1960s.

It is significant to note that Paoli has reached a similar conclusion, although she has a very different starting point from that taken here and she uses very different methods, a different framework and different data sources. Paoli is a criminologist who, on the basis of her work in the area of drug use in sport, was invited to chair the *Evaluierungskommission Freiburger Sportmedizin*, which investigated the role of sports physicians at Freiburg University in the doping of German athletes since the 1950s. Paoli's research has focused primarily on the investigation of the structure of the market – and particularly the supply side of the market – for performance-enhancing drugs. Based on a detailed analysis of the market for performance-enhancing drugs in Italy, France and Belgium, as well as her work as Chair of the Freiburg Commission, Paoli concludes that physicians 'have … been repeatedly active as suppliers of doping products in the elite segment of the market', and that this trend 'is part of the broader involvement of physicians in the treatment of elite athletes since World War II' (Paoli, 2019: 83).

In the next chapter, we provide three detailed case studies of the involvement of sports physicians in doping. Two of these case studies can perhaps be best understood in terms of the way in which the role of the sports physician has been affected by the politicisation of sport, while two of the cases examine the role of sports physicians not merely in the prescribing or provision of drugs to athletes, but in the actual *development* of drugs and doping techniques specifically with a view to enhancing athletic performance.

References

Armstrong, R. (1991), Anti-doping procedures and legal consequences. Medical and ethical factors and conflicts of interest, in International Athletic Foundation, International Symposium on Sport and Law: Official Proceedings. International Athletic Foundation, Monte Carlo, Monaco.

British Medical Association (BMA) (1996), *Sport and Exercise Medicine: Policy and Provision*, London, BMA.

Clarke, A. E., Mamo, L., Fishman, J. R., Shim, J. K. and Fosket, J. F. (2003), Biomedicalisation: technoscientific transformations of health, illness, and U.S. biomedicine, *American Sociological Review*, 68, 161–194.

Coni, P., Kelland, G. and Davies, D. (1988), *AAA Drug Abuse Enquiry Report*, Birmingham, Amateur Athletics Association

Conrad, P. (2005), The shifting engines of medicalization, *Journal of Health and Social Behavior*, 46 , 3–14.

De Swaan, A. (1988), *In Care of the State*, Cambridge, Cambridge University Press.

Dennis, M. (2015), The East German doping programme, in V. Møller, I. Waddington and J. Hoberman (eds), *Routledge Handbook of Drugs and Sport*, Abingdon, Routledge, 170–180.

Donati, A. (2004), The silent drama of the diffusion of doping among amateurs and professionals, in J. Hoberman and V. Moller (eds), *Doping and Public Policy*, Odense, University of Southern Denmark.

Donati, A. (2006), Doping and doping control in Italian sport, in G. Spitzer (ed), *Doping and Doping Control in Europe,* Oxford, Meyer and Meyer

Donlan, L. (2014) An empirical assessment of factors affecting the brand-building effectiveness of sponsors. *Sport, Business and Management: An International Journal*, 4 (1), 6–25.

Donohoe, T. and Johnson, N. (1986), *Foul Play: Drug Abuse in Sports*, Oxford, Blackwell.

Dubin, The Hon Charles L. (1990), *Commission of Inquiry into the Use of Drugs and Banned Practices Intended to Increase Athletic Performance*, Ottawa, Canadian Government Publishing Centre.

FIMS (2023) www.fims.org Accessed 7 June 2023

Gough, C. (2024), Sports sponsorship - statistics and facts, https://www.statista.com/topics /1382/sports-sponsorship Accessed 16 May 2024.

Gratton, C. and Taylor, P. (2000). *The Economics of Sport and Recreation*, London, Routledge.

Guttmann, A. (1992), *The Olympics: A History of the Modern Games,* Urbana and Chicago, University of Illinois Press.

Hamilton, T. and Coyle, D. (2012), *The Secret Race*, London, Bantam Press.

Heggie, V. (2011), *A History of British Sports Medicine*, Manchester, Manchester University Press.

Hill, C. (1992), *Olympic Politics*, Manchester, Manchester University Press.

Hoberman, J. (1992), The early development of sports medicine in Germany, in J. W. Berryman and R. J. Park (eds), *Sport and Exercise Science: Essays in the History of Sports Medicine*, Urbana and Chicago, University of Illinois Press, 233–282.

Houlihan, B. (2002), *Dying to Win: Doping in Sport and the Development of Anti-Doping Policy*, 2nd ed., Strasbourg, Council of Europe.

Illich, I. (1975), *Medical Nemesis*, London, Calder and Boyars.

Laure, P. (1997), Doping in sport: doctors are providing drugs, *British Journal of Sports Medicine*, 31, 258–259.

Luschen, G. (2000), Doping in sport as deviant behaviour and its social control, in J.Coakley and E. Dunning (eds), *Handbook of Sports Studies*, London, Sage, 461–476.

Malcolm, D. (2017), *Sport, Medicine and Health*, London, Routledge.

Mandell, R. (1987), *The Nazi Olympics*, Urbana and Chicago, University of Illinois Press.

On the Line (1990), Drugs, lies and finishing tape, *BBC2 TV*, 24 January.

Paoli, L. (2019), The peculiarities of the role of the market for doping products and the role of academic physicians, in B. Fincoeur, J. Gleaves and F. Ohl (eds), *Doping in Cycling: Interdisciplinary Perspectives*, London, Routledge, 79–96.

Paoli, L. and Donati, A. (2014), *The Sports Doping Market: Understanding Supply and Demand and the Challenges of Their Control*, New York, Springer.

Roberts, R. and Olsen, J. (1989), *Winning is the Only Thing,* Baltimore, MD, Johns Hopkins University Press.

Safai, P. (2007), A critical analysis of the development of sport medicine in Canada, 1955–1980, *International Review for the Sociology of Sport*, 42 (3), 321–341.

Sperryn, P. (1983), *Sport and Medicine*, London, Butterworth.

Todd, J. and Todd, T. (2001), Significant events in the history of drug testing and the Olympic movement: 1960–99, in W. Wilson and E. Derse (eds), *Doping in Elite Sport*, Champaign, IL, Human Kinetics.

Verroken, M. (2005), Drug use and abuse in sport, in D. Mottram (ed.) *Drugs in Sport*, 4th ed. London, Routledge.

Voy, R. (1991), *Drugs, Sport and Politics*, Champaign, IL, Leisure Press.

Waddington, I. (2000), *Sport, Health and Drugs*, London, Spon.

Waddington, I. and Smith, A. (2009), *An Introduction to Drugs in Sport: Addicted to Winning?* London, Routledge.

Waitzkin, H. and Waterman, B. (1974), *The Exploitation of Illness in Capitalist Society*, New York, Bobbs-Merrill.

Williams, J. G. P. (1962), *Sports Medicine*, London, Edward Arnold.
Williams, J. G. P. and Sperryn, P. (eds) (1976), *Sports Medicine*, 2nd ed., London, Edward Arnold.
Yesalis, C. E. and and Bahrke, M. S. (2005), Anabolic steroid and stimulant use in North American Sport between 1850 and 1980, *Sport in History*, 25 (3), 434–451.
Zola, I. (1972), Medicine as an instrument of social control, *Sociological Review*, 20, 487–504.

7 Sports medicine and the development and use of performance-enhancing drugs

Three case studies

We noted in Chapter 3 that the work of early physiologists who carried out experiments on athletes was not concerned with boosting athletic performance, but simply with developing a better understanding of how the human body works. As we saw in Chapter 4, this orientation began to change in Germany from the 1920s, when the DÄB, headed by the physician and former Olympic athlete Mallwitz and supported by the German Olympic Association, made the decisive shift towards an emphasis on high-level competitive sport and towards improving the performances of German athletes, a process which, as we saw, also involved some of the leading German sports physicians of the time in the search for performance-enhancing drugs. In this regard, as in many others, German sports physicians led where others followed. In more recent years, and particularly in the post-1945 period, the increased emphasis which has come to be placed on winning and on breaking records has dramatically changed the relationship between athletic performance and sports medicine in almost all societies which have elite-level athletes competing in international competitions.

It is important to stress that the increased involvement of sports physicians in the search for enhanced athletic performance has involved a radical shift in the research orientation of sports medicine and, associated with this, an equally dramatic change in the nature of sports medicine as a discipline. This process has involved a shift away from the situation in which sports physicians, in the late nineteenth and early twentieth centuries, saw sport primarily as a source of data for the study of human physiology and were more or less uninterested in enhancing sporting performance and the attempt to set new athletic records; conversely, as sports physicians have become more and more involved in a sporting world which, particularly in the post-1945 period, has become increasingly competitive, so have their scientific activities both increasingly underpinned, and increasingly been given meaning by, the search for enhanced athletic performances. If the late nineteenth and early twentieth century pioneers of sports medicine were largely unconcerned about improving athletic performance, this has now become an important part of the raison d'être of contemporary sports medicine. And we have argued that one particularly problematic aspect of the search for enhanced performances has been the growing involvement of sports physicians in the development and use of use of banned substances and techniques.

DOI: 10.4324/9781003563921-10

Sports medicine and drugs

A more-or-less standard feature of modern textbooks on sports medicine is the inclusion of a chapter on the use of performance-enhancing drugs. Such chapters usually include basic information on the performance-enhancing effects of different drugs, on the side-effects and other medical complications which may be associated with their use, and advice to physicians on how to recognise the illicit use of drugs by athletes under their care. Associated with the inclusion of information of this kind in textbooks of sports medicine is the public perception of the practitioner of sports medicine as an expert who plays a vital role in the fight against what is commonly described as the 'abuse' of drugs in sport. However, the analysis in the previous chapter suggests that the relationship between the development of sports medicine and the development and use of performance-enhancing drugs is a good deal more complex than is usually presented in textbooks of sports medicine. In particular, such an analysis suggests that the growing involvement of practitioners of sports medicine in elite sport from the 1950s – and more particularly in the search for enhanced sporting performances – has increasingly led them in the direction not only of developing improved diet or mechanical and psychological techniques but that, on occasions, it has also led them – though it is not suggested that they have always been aware of the longer-term consequences of their actions – to play an active part in the development and use of performance-enhancing drugs. Thus it is suggested that, far from being one of the key bastions in the fight against the use of performance-enhancing drugs in sport, sports medicine has actually been one of the major contexts within which performance-enhancing drugs have been developed and used. In this sense, it may be said that *the development of performance-enhancing drugs and techniques is not something which is alien to, but something which has been an integral part of, the recent history of sports medicine.* This aspect of the development of sports medicine will be explored further *via* an examination of three illustrative case studies: the relationship between sports medicine and the use of drugs in some of the former communist countries of Eastern Europe; the early development and use of anabolic steroids in the United States; and the development of the technique which has come to be known as 'blood doping'. The first case study highlights the very complex structure of state-sponsored doping programmes (a structure which was recently replicated in the Russian state-sponsored doping system [Mclaren, 2016a, 2016b]). The other two cases highlight a key aspect of Elias's approach to sociology, namely his focus on unplanned outcomes, that is to say that the very complex nature of the networks of relationships in which we are involved means that very frequently our actions have consequences which we did not intend and which we may well not have wanted.

Sports medicine and drug use in Eastern Europe

The proportion of Olympic medals won by athletes from Eastern European communist countries increased dramatically from 29 per cent in 1952 to 57 per cent in 1976 (Malcolm, 2017: 41) and, for many years prior to the collapse of the communist regimes in Eastern Europe, there were widespread suspicions among western observers that the outstanding successes of many East European, and particularly East German and Soviet, athletes were associated, at least in part, with the use of performance-enhancing drugs. Since the collapse of those regimes, very much more information has become available, and we now know that performance-enhancing drugs were used systematically by those involved in the sports medical establishments of some Soviet bloc countries in their attempt to produce Olympic medal-winning athletes.

It would be very misleading to suggest that the successes of East German and Soviet athletes can simply be explained in terms of the use of performance-enhancing drugs, for in both countries there was a well-developed system for talent-screening, while all aspects of the training and development of elite athletes were carefully monitored by sports physicians who worked within a highly sophisticated system of sports medicine (Spitzer, 2004, 2006a). Nevertheless, it is clear that the systematic use of drugs was an integral part of the sport systems in several East European communist countries.

In relation to the situation in the former Soviet Union, Riordan has noted that:

> It should come as no surprise that, given the 'win at all costs' mentality that came to dominate the sports administrations in some East European countries, there had been long-term *state* production, testing, monitoring and administering of performance-enhancing drugs in regard to athletes as young as 7-8.
> (Riordan, 1994, emphasis in original)

Elsewhere, Riordan (1991: 122) has suggested that practices such as this have cast 'a shadow over the role of sports medicine, or at least that part of it that has worked on producing ever faster, stronger, more skilful athletes – at any cost'.

There is, perhaps, no need to document in detail the multiplicity of ways in which, we now know, members of the sports medicine establishments in the Soviet Union and East Germany were involved in the use of performance-enhancing drugs. What is important to note is that the use of such drugs was a systematic part of sport policy in the Soviet Union and East Germany, and that it involved a wide variety of people, including sports physicians, the 'coach-pharmacologist' and government ministers. As Riordan has noted in relation to the Soviet Union:

> Drug taking was organised *at the top* and involved parts of the sports medical establishment; no athlete was allowed overseas unless he or she had a clearance test at a sports medicine dispensary before departure. At the Olympics of Montreal (1976) and Seoul (1988), it has now been revealed, the Soviet team had a hospitality ship used as a medical centre to ensure that Soviet competitors were 'clean' at the last moment.
> (Riordan, 1991: 123: emphases in original)

A similar system, which also involved sports physicians, operated in communist Czechoslovakia (Waddington and Smith, 2009: 91).

However, the most highly developed state-sponsored doping programme was undoubtedly that which was developed in East Germany and which helped that country to become, in terms of Olympic medals, the world's most successful sporting nation per head of population; at its last appearance at a major event, the 1998 summer Olympics, East Germany, with a population of just over 17 million, finished second in the unofficial medals table (Dennis, 2015: 170). Documents which have become available since the fall of the Communist regime in East Germany indicate that an estimated 2,000 athletes, seniors as well as juniors, were 'doped' each year from about 1972 (Dennis, 2015: 170). In total, in the period up to the collapse of East Germany in 1989–90, drugs were administered to an estimated 10,000 male and female athletes, often without their knowledge or consent, while two million doses of anabolic steroids were used annually in the preparation for Olympic sports (Spitzer, 2006b: 109).

The administration of performance-enhancing drugs to athletes involved personnel in a number of organisations, including the German College of Physical Culture, the Research Institute for Physical Culture and Sport, the Central Institute for Microbiology and Experimental Therapy, the pharmaceutical company VEB Jenapharm, the Central Institute for Sports Medical Services, the Central Doping-Control Laboratory in Kreischa, the Institute for Aviation Medicine and the Health Ministry in East Berlin (Hoberman, 1992: 222). Sports physicians were central to the operation of this system, *which involved at least 700 doctors and other medical personnel* in the Sports Medical Service (Dennis, 2015: 170). At the apex of this system was Dr Manfred Höppner, the leading sports physician in East Germany, who headed two groups which were pivotal to the scheme: the 'Central Work Group on Supportive Means' and the 'Research Group on Supportive Means'. The former, established in 1975 as part of the Sports Medical Service high-performance sector, oversaw the distribution of drugs to sports physicians, trainers and athletes (Dennis, 2015: 173). It is significant that the euphemism used for drugs in East Germany – 'supportive means' – was, as we saw in Chapter 4, very similar to the euphemism ('Hilfe') used by German doctors who were involved in experiments with performance-enhancing drugs in the 1920s and 1930s, and as we shall see in Chapter 9, it was also very similar to the euphemisms used by French sports physicians in the 1960s.

Physicians in the state-run Sports Medical Service were involved in determining the doping guidelines for a four-year period, while doctors in the individual sports federations administered the doping substances according to central guidelines. As Spitzer (2006a: 124) has noted, the 'pursuit of sporting excellence was the objective of sport scientists, physicians and biologists, even if this meant breaching … the conventional understanding of medical ethics'. Clear breaches of medical ethics included administering drugs to athletes without their knowledge or consent; withholding information from athletes about the known side-effects, especially on women, of very high doses of anabolic steroids; falsifying athletes' health data following their retirement from athletics; and doping children, some as young as ten years old (Spitzer, 2001, 2006b). Doctors were expected to practise in what Spitzer has described as a 'hard line' manner; those who were 'more oriented towards the welfare of athletes were removed from the system and relocated into the general medical service' (Spitzer, 2006b: 122).

It is important to emphasise that the use of drugs by Soviet and East German athletes was not something which was done against the advice of, or without the knowledge and consent of, those involved in the sports federations and in the sports medicine establishments of those countries; rather it is the case that the drugs were provided by the state, and that all aspects of the athletes' development, *including those relating to the administration of drugs, were supervised and monitored by specialists in sports medicine.* Within the context of sport in some of the former communist regimes of Eastern Europe, therefore, it is not possible to separate out the development and use of performance-enhancing drugs from the development of sports medicine, for the one was an integral part of the other. The use of performance-enhancing drugs was viewed simply as one part of the scientific armoury which also included such things as diet, exercise physiology and biomechanics, and which was available to sports physicians in their efforts to produce medal-winning athletes.

Malcolm (2017: 42) has described the situation in the Soviet Union and East Germany during this period as one which involved 'the alignment of sports medicine with nationalist goals'. That this phenomenon was not limited to Eastern European communist states is clearly illustrated by the following case study.

The development and use of anabolic steroids in the United States

In the early 1950s there were persistent rumours among western athletes to the effect that sports physicians in the Soviet Union had been carrying out experiments with testosterone in an attempt to boost the performances of Soviet athletes. According to Voy (1991), positive confirmation of these rumours came at the 1956 World Games in Moscow, when Dr John Ziegler, who was the team physician to the United States team, witnessed urinary catheters being used by Soviet male athletes. Ziegler was not surprised by this, for he knew that the use of testosterone would enlarge the prostate, possibly to the point where the urinary tract would be obstructed, thus making it difficult for the athletes to urinate. Because of this, athletes sometimes used urinary catheters in order to facilitate urination (Voy, 1991).

On returning to the United States, Ziegler obtained some testosterone and tested it on himself, on the US weightlifting coach, Bob Hoffman, and on several east coast weightlifters. Ziegler was impressed by the anabolic, or muscle-building, effects of testosterone but concerned about some of the side-effects. According to Voy:

> In an attempt to help Western athletes compete more effectively against the Soviets who used testosterone, and in an effort to reduce the bad side effects of testosterone – namely, acne, hair loss, prostate enlargement, and shrinkage of the testicles – Dr Ziegler aided the CIBA Pharmaceutical Company in the development of Dianabol, or, in generic terms, methandrostenolone.
>
> (Voy, 1991: 9)

As developed by CIBA, the drug was not intended for use by athletes, but was developed for use in treating patients suffering from burns and certain post-operative patients. However, as Todd (1987: 94) has noted, Dr Ziegler 'had another agenda, and what he did with Dianabol was critical in the spread of anabolic drugs in sport'. With the cooperation of the national weightlifting coach, Ziegler persuaded three weightlifters to begin using Dianabol. Almost immediately, the three lifters began making very rapid gains in strength and muscle size and, as the lifters began to approach the world record level, other lifters clamoured for information about how this rapid improvement had been achieved. It soon became widely known that the success of the three lifters, by this time all national champions, had been associated with their use of Dianabol. According to Voy (1991), Dianabol was among the first 'big time' anabolic-androgenic steroids and its use spread rapidly among American athletes: indeed, anabolic steroids were adopted so quickly by American athletes that it was estimated that by 1968, a full third of the US track and field team had used steroids at the pre-Olympic training camp held at Lake Tahoe, prior to the Mexico Olympics (Todd, 1987: 95). In the 1980s, Dianabol was used by Ben Johnson and by other athletes who were coached by Charlie Francis, including Angela Issajenko (Dubin, 1990: 244–246).

As both Voy and Todd recognise, Ziegler played a central role in helping to produce 'a climate of rising expectations in which strength athletes began a big arms race, fuelled by an ever expanding array of pharmaceuticals' (Todd, 1987: 94).[1] In the mid-1980s, the central role of Ziegler in the development and use of anabolic steroids was recognised, with wonderful irony, in the name of a California-based business which supplied athletes with steroids by mail-order; the business was called the John Ziegler Fan Club (Todd, 1987: 104).

As we noted earlier, it is not suggested that sports physicians who have become involved in the search for performance-enhancing drugs have always been fully aware of the longer-term consequences of their actions, for their actions, like all human actions, are constrained by a complex network of relationships of which they are likely to have, at best, only a limited awareness. In the case of Dr Ziegler, Voy (1991: 10) has pointed out that, particularly when he became aware of the high doses being taken by some athletes, Ziegler:

> realized the mistake he had made by helping to introduce these drugs to the athletic community. It was almost a sports world analogy to the story of Dr Frankenstein. Soon after Dianabol hit the market, Dr Ziegler knew he had created a monster, a fact he regretted for the rest of his life.

It is important to emphasise that it is not possible to dismiss Ziegler simply as a charlatan, as a disreputable practitioner on the fringes of, or even outside of, orthodox sports medicine. Nor is it possible to dismiss Ziegler as a cheat whose actions ran counter to the rules of fair play; in this context it is important to emphasise that in the 1950s and early 1960s, taking pills to enhance performance was not against the rules of any sporting competition, for there were no anti-doping regulations at that time. This was a period, it should be recalled, when more effective drugs – most notably antibiotics – were becoming available to doctors in their treatment of patients, and when patients were also becoming more aware of the therapeutic possibilities offered by new drugs. America was, as Voy puts it, 'a society that was just developing the pill-popping scene' and, within this context, it is not surprising that both sports physicians and athletes should have looked to the pharmaceutical industry to improve athletic performances, just as it held out the possibility of improving many other aspects of people's lives. In this sense, Ziegler's actions should be seen not as those of an idiosyncratic zealot, nor as the actions of a disreputable cheat, but simply as the actions of a sports physician whose involvement in the increasingly competitive world of modern sport led him, just as it led other sports physicians, towards the search for performance-enhancing drugs.

Of course, it might be objected that both case studies cited above are atypical and that, as a consequence, they cannot be regarded as shedding much light on the more general relationship between the development of sports medicine and the search for, and the use of, performance-enhancing drugs. It might, for example, be argued that the case of sports medicine in Eastern Europe related to totalitarian communist regimes which, in one sense or another, were 'abnormal', which can therefore shed little light on the development of sports medicine in the liberal democracies of the West and which, in any case, no longer exist. In similar fashion, it might be objected that the case study of the development of Dianabol, though relating to a liberal democracy, also relates to a period when there were no rules prohibiting the use of performance-enhancing drugs and when the situation was therefore very different from that which exists today, where there are relatively clear rules which prohibit the use of such drugs; on this basis, it might be objected that the situation described in relation to the development of Dianabol was merely an 'unfortunate', one-off incident and not one which would be likely to be repeated today. In the context of possible objections of this kind, the third case study – the development of the technique which has come to be known as 'blood doping' – is particularly revealing.

Blood doping

Blood doping does not involve the administration of drugs, but is a technique involving the removal from an athlete of some blood, which is stored and later reinfused into the athlete. The removal of this blood stimulates the bone marrow to form more red cells, and the athlete's blood returns to normal after 10–12 weeks. The stored blood is then reinfused into the athlete a couple of days before competition, the extra red cells boosting the oxygen-carrying capacity of the blood, and thus the quantity of oxygen available to the muscles.

Although some early work on blood doping had been done in the 1940s, the technique did not become associated with sport until many years later. The first systematic research studies to examine the effects of blood doping on endurance and performance were conducted in Sweden, during the late 1960s and early 1970s, by Professor Bjorn Ekblom and his colleagues at the Institute of Physiology of Performance in Stockholm. They initially reported significant increases in maximum oxygen uptake and went on to claim that blood doping was associated with significant improvements in performance (Donohoe and Johnson, 1986: 116–117). In the 1970s and early 1980s many similar studies were undertaken by sports physicians and related specialists within sports medicine with a view to discovering whether blood doping was indeed an effective means of improving performance. Although there were some contradictory findings from the early studies, by the early 1980s a consensus of opinion was emerging to the effect that, carried out in the appropriate way, blood doping was indeed an effective way of increasing maximum oxygen uptake and endurance capacity (Williams, 1981; Gledhill, 1982). A review of the contradictory findings from earlier studies also led to considerable refinements in the technique of blood doping. Thus, for example, it was suggested that the failure of some of the early studies to find a significant improvement in performance following reinfusion was associated with the use of inadequate reinfusion volumes, or with premature reinfusion of blood following removal or with inappropriate methods of storing the blood. Sports physicians were thus able to indicate that, for the maximum impact in terms of improving athletic performance, a specified minimal amount of blood should be reinfused, there should be a specified minimum interval between removal of the blood and reinfusion, and that the blood should be stored by freezing rather than by refrigeration in order to avoid the loss of red cells in the blood (Gledhill, 1982).

Outside the world of sports medicine, there had been some popular interest in blood doping in the 1970s when some commentators suggested that the Finnish runner Lasse Viren, a double gold medallist at both the 1972 and 1976 Olympics, had been blood doped; Viren vigorously denied the suggestion and attributed his success to drinking reindeer milk. Media and popular interest in the technique was revived when, following the spectacular success of the US cycling team at the Los Angeles Olympics in 1984 – the United States, which had not won an Olympic cycling medal since 1912, dominated the cycling events at the 1984 Games, winning a total of nine medals, including four gold – it was revealed that several members of the US team had been blood doped (Cramer, 1985; Pavelka, 1985; Weaver, 1985). Following these revelations, the IOC declared the practice illegal and funded research into the development of methods for detecting blood doping (Collings, 1988).

In considering the development of the technique of blood doping from the early 1970s, it should be noted that the research which demonstrated that blood doping was an effective method of boosting athletic performance and which also led to considerable refinements of that technique – thus improving its effectiveness as a means of boosting performance – was carried out by sports physicians and related specialists within sports medicine. It is important to emphasise that those involved in this research were not those who might be regarded as 'quacks', working on the illegitimate fringes of sports medicine and rejected by their more reputable colleagues, but that they were highly reputable sports physicians working within the mainstream of sports medicine, and their research was published, not in underground publications which circulated illicitly, but in the mainstream journals in sports medicine.

Viewed sociologically, what one might call the 'moral career' of blood doping is very interesting for, within two decades, what had formerly been regarded as a legitimate research area for sports physicians seeking to improve athletic performance came to be regarded as a form of cheating which was banned under the anti-doping rules of the IOC. A brief examination of the shift in the status of blood doping, from legitimate to illegitimate technique, is particularly revealing in terms of understanding the relationship between sports medicine and the use of performance-enhancing drugs and techniques.

An examination of the early literature on blood doping suggests that sports physicians initially regarded blood doping simply as one of many science-based techniques, such as diet or biometric analysis, which held out the possibility of boosting athletic performance and that, at least in these early stages, they had little awareness of the possibility that its use might be construed as a form of cheating. For example, in one of the early major British textbooks, *Sports Medicine*, by JGP Williams and PN Sperryn (1976), there was just one brief reference to blood doping, which was as follows:

> Experimental re-transfusion of subjects with their own red cells after an interval of four weeks was thought to give improved performance, but this has subsequently been denied by further studies. In view of the dangers inherent in the whole process of blood transfusion, it is unlikely that further developments can be expected.
>
> (1976: 158)

We need not concern ourselves here with the inaccuracy of their forecast about future developments; what is of interest is the absence of any suggestion that such a technique might be construed as cheating. This is confirmed by the fact that the discussion of blood doping is located, not in the chapter on doping, but in a chapter entitled 'General medical aspects of sport'. Within this chapter, the brief discussion of blood doping is located in a section on 'Hazards of exercise' which deals with such things as general medical screening, inoculations, routine clinical examinations, physiological testing, infections, sex and skin disorders. One can only conclude that Williams and Sperryn considered it appropriate to discuss blood doping under the heading 'General medical aspects of sport' and that they saw no reason to include it in their discussion of doping. This would suggest that they regarded it as a legitimate area for research and development – even if, in their view, it was an unpromising development – for practitioners of sports medicine.

Seven years later, Sperryn's *Sport and Medicine* (1983) included a slightly expanded discussion of blood doping, but there was still no suggestion that blood doping might be construed as a form of cheating. After a brief discussion of some of the technical aspects of blood doping, Sperryn concludes:

> In summary, while this method is theoretically attractive, its practice must be extremely difficult to regulate safely and efficiently under all the stresses of athletic competition and, in view of all the provisos outlined, it is unlikely to become widespread.
>
> (1983: 27)

Again we are not concerned with whether or not Sperryn's prediction about the use of blood doping was correct – this was, it might be noted, just one year before the

United States cycling team used the technique to such good effect – but with the absence of any suggestion that the use of the technique could be considered a form of cheating. In this context, Sperryn rejects the technique not because he considers its use runs counter to the spirit of 'fair play', but because of certain technical difficulties in using it 'under all the stresses of athletic competition'. It is once again significant that this discussion of blood doping is located not in the chapter on doping in Sperryn's book but, on this occasion, in a chapter on 'Cardiovascular and respiratory systems'. Given the date of publication of Sperryn's book, it is perhaps surprising that he made no reference to any ethical issues in his discussion of blood doping for, by the late 1970s and early 1980s, sports physicians were increasingly raising the question of whether the technique which they themselves had pioneered might not give rise to ethical concerns relating to concepts of fairness and cheating. However, it should be emphasised that, particularly in the 1970s, most researchers appeared to be as unconcerned with ethical issues as were Williams and Sperryn. It might be noted that two research papers on blood doping which did explicitly raise ethical issues were those by Videman and Rytömaa (1977) and by Williams, Lindhjem and Schuster (1978). However, in both cases, the ethical issues which were discussed related not to fair play and cheating, but to the rather different ethical issues, such as those relating to informed consent, which are raised when using human subjects in experimental programmes.

By the late 1970s and early 1980s, however, it was becoming increasingly common for researchers to discuss not only the technical aspects of blood doping, but also to raise the question of whether or not blood doping could be regarded as a form of cheating (Gledhill, 1982; Gledhill and Froese, 1979; Williams, 1981). Writers at the time seemed to see this as a difficult issue to resolve, not least because a similar effect to that obtained by blood doping could also be obtained by training at altitude, a practice which was allowed – and still is allowed; indeed, how could it be banned? – by all sports governing bodies (Gledhill and Froese, 1979: 25). Williams concluded his brief discussion of ethical issues by calling on the governing bodies of sport to consider the matter:

> Because it is an effective method of improving distance running performance, its place in the sports world should be determined by the various governing bodies.
>
> (Williams, 1981: 61)

By this time, it is clear that the status of blood doping was changing. From being a technique which, in the early 1970s, raised technical issues but not, for most researchers, issues of fairness, it had become a technique the ethical status of which was now uncertain. It was not yet, however, unambiguously regarded as a form of cheating.

The final stage in the 'moral career' of blood doping came with the decision by the IOC, following the 1984 Olympic Games, to ban the practice of blood doping. Once the IOC had taken this decision, the view that blood doping was a form of cheating quickly became established as the orthodoxy among practitioners of sports medicine. Thus in 1987, the American College of Sports Medicine issued a 'position stand', in which it stated: 'It is the position of the American College of Sports Medicine that the use of blood doping as an ergogenic aid for athletic competition is unethical and unjustifiable' (1987: 540). The following year Dirix, writing in *The Olympic Book of Sports Medicine*, held that the procedures involved in blood doping 'contravene the ethics of medicine and of sport' (1988: 674). There was, it is true, still the occasional sceptical view, such as that expressed in 1988 by Nuzzo and Waller, who reminded their readers that training at high altitude can lead to an increase in red blood cells (RBC), and suggested that this could place athletes trained at low altitude at a disadvantage. They then went on to ask: 'Should blood doping be permitted to make all competitors have equal RBC concentrations?' (1988: 148). By this time, however, such views were rare. Much more common was the view expressed by Eriksson and his colleagues (1990: 383) and by Cowan (1994: 327), who not only echoed the sentiment which had earlier been expressed by Dirix, but also used his precise words: 'These procedures contravene the ethics of medicine and of sport'. Mottram (1988: 23) similarly held that 'Apart from contravening the ethics of sport and medicine, this procedure carries tremendous risk to the individual recipient'. MacAuley (1991: 83), writing in a book published for the Sports Council for Northern Ireland, described the technique of blood doping and then noted: 'It is of course banned', as though the technique were so self-evidently a form of cheating that it was difficult to see how this issue could ever have been problematic. Rather more sophisticated was the position of Wadler and Hainline, who argued that blood doping 'is unique in that the inability to detect its use, coupled with its clear-cut ergogenic potential, demands from the individual athlete a more profound ethical and moral decision. As with other drugs and methods of deception which are always available, the athlete is left with a choice – to embrace the meaning of the essence of sport, or to participate in the practice of winning at any cost' (1989: 176). The argument may have been a little more sophisticated, but the message was the same: blood doping is cheating.

By the late 1980s, then, a new moral orthodoxy in relation to blood doping had been established. By this time, sports physicians, acting not merely as technical experts but also as moral 'police' charged with the responsibility of educating athletes about both the ethics and the medical dangers of using banned substances or techniques, were telling athletes in unambiguous terms that the use of blood doping was cheating and that this technique should not be used. It is a reasonable supposition that, when advising athletes in their care, they did not tell the athletes that it was they – the sports physicians – who had developed and refined this technique. It is not perhaps surprising that, within this context, sports physicians chose to ignore certain aspects of the history of blood doping. Thus Goldman and Klatz, in their *Death in the Locker Room II*, wrote in relation to blood doping that 'Some athletes will go to any length to boost their endurance and performance' (1992: 203). The implication of their statement would seem to be that, if anyone is culpable in relation to the use of blood doping, then it is the athletes. One might easily get the impression from Goldman that it was the athletes themselves, rather than Goldman's own colleagues within sports medicine, who had developed the technique.

Conclusion

The close interrelationship between sports medicine and the development of what have come to be regarded as illicit drugs and techniques was nicely brought out by Cramer in his report on the use of blood doping by the United States cycling team at the 1984 Olympics:

> In the national euphoria after the games, no one thought to pry out any secrets. The US team had won nine medals, dominating the cycling events. 'Great riders …' 'Great coach …' 'Great bikes …' said the press, reporting the daisy chain of back pats. No one thought to add, 'Great doctors'.
>
> (1985: 25)

An important implication of the case studies discussed above, as well as the data about medical involvement in doping presented in the previous chapter, is that if we wish to understand the processes involved in the increase from the 1960s in the illicit use by elite athletes of performance-enhancing drugs, then we need to shift our focus away from what has usually been an almost exclusive concentration on the drug-using athletes, and to examine more closely the networks of relationships in which athletes are involved (Waddington, 2019; Waddington and Møller, 2019). Clearly, one aspect of this must involve a much closer, and more critical, examination of the relationships between athletes and sports physicians.

Note

1 Note Todd's clever play on words with his use of the phrase 'big arms race', which correctly locates the sporting competition between the United States and the Soviet Union in the context of the Cold War and superpower rivalry.

References

American College of Sports Medicine (1987), American College of Sports Medicine position stand on blood doping as an ergogenic aid, *Medicine and Science in Sports and Exercise*, 19, 540–543.

Collings, A. F. (1988), Blood doping: how, why and why not, *Excel* (Canberra, AC), 4, 12–16.

Cowan, D. A. (1994), Drug abuse, in M. Harries, C. Williams, W. D. Standish and L. J. Micheli (eds), *Oxford Textbook of Sports Medicine*, Oxford, Oxford University Press.

Cramer, R. B. (1985), Olympic cheating: the inside story of illicit doping and the US cycling team, *Rolling Stone*, 441, 25–26, 30.

Dennis, M. (2015), The East German doping programme, in V. Møller, I. Waddington and J. M. Hoberman (eds), *The Routledge Handbook of Drugs and Sport*, Abingdon, Routledge, 170–180

Dirix, A. (1988), Classes and methods, in A. Dirix, H. G. Knuttgen and K. Tittel (eds), *The Olympic Book of Sports Medicine,* Oxford, Blackwell.

Donohoe, T. and Johnson, N. (1986), *Foul Play: Drug Abuse in Sports*, Oxford, Blackwell.

Dubin, The Hon. Charles L. (1990), *Commission of Inquiry into the Use of Drugs and Banned Practices Intended to Increase Athletic Performance*, Ottawa, Canadian Government Publishing Centre.

Eriksson, B. O., Mellstrand, T., Peterson, L. and Renström, P. (1990), *Sports Medicine*, Enfield, Guinness Publishing.

Gledhill, N. (1982), Blood doping and related issues: a brief review, *Medicine and Science in Sport and Exercise*, 14, 183–189.

Gledhill, N. and Froese, A. (1979), Should research on blood doping be continued? *Modern Athlete and Coach*, 17, 23–25.

Goldman, B. and Klatz, R. (1992), *Death in the Locker Room II*, Chicago, Elite Sports Medicine Publications.

Hoberman. J. (1992), *Mortal Engines: The Science of Performance and the Dehumanization of Sport,* New York, Free Press.

MacAuley, D. (1991), *Sports Medicine*, Northern Ireland: Quest Books (N.I.) for the Sports Council of Northern Ireland.

Mclaren, R. H. (2016a), *Independent Person Report: WADA Investigation of Sochi Allegations.* Montreal, WADA.

Mclaren, R. H. (2016b), *Independent Person 2nd Report: WADA Investigation of Sochi Allegations*. Montreal, WADA.

Malcolm, D. (2017), *Sport. Medicine and Health*, London, Routledge.

Mottram, D. (1988), Drugs in Sport, London, E & F N Spon.

Nuzzo, N. and Waller, D (1988), Drug abuse in athletes, in J. Thomas (ed.), *Drugs, Athletes and Physical Performance*, London and New York, Plenum Medical Books Co.

Pavelka, E. (1985), Olympic blood boosting: How American cyclists sweated blood – literally – to win, *Bicycling* (Emmaus, Pa), April, 32–39.

Riordan, J. (1991), *Sport, Politics and Communism*, Manchester, Manchester University Press.

Riordan, J. (1994), The use of ergogenic aids in Eastern Europe: Ethics and ethos, paper presented to the 1994 IOC Sports Medicine Course, Hong Kong Sports Institute, March.

Sperryn, P. (1983), *Sport and Medicine*, London, Butterworth.

Spitzer, G. (2001), Doping with children, in C. Peters, T. Schulz and H. Michna (eds), *Biomedical Side Effects of Doping*, Bonn, Bundesinstitut für Sportwissenschaft.

Spitzer, G. (2004), A Leninist monster: compulsory doping and public policy in the GDR and the lessons for today, in J. Hoberman and V. Møller (eds), *Doping and Public Policy*, Odense, University Press of Southern Denmark, 133–143.

Spitzer, G. (2006a), Ranking number 3 in the world: how the addiction to doping changed sport in the GDR, in G. Spitzer (ed.), *Doping and Doping Control in Europe*, Aachen, Meyer and Meyer, 57–77.

Spitzer, G. (2006b), Sport and the systematic infliction of pain: a case study of state-sponsored mandatory doping in East Germany, in S. Loland, B. Skirstad and I. Waddington (eds), *Pain and Injury in Sport*, London, Routledge, 109–126.

Todd, T. (1987), Anabolic steroids: the gremlins of sport, *Journal of Sport History*, 14, 87–107.

Videman, T. and Rytomaa, T. (1977), Effect of blood removal and autotransfusion on heart rate response to a submaximal workload, *Journal of Sports Medicine*, 17, 387–390.

Voy, R. (1991), *Drugs, Sport and Politics*, Champaign, IL, Leisure Press.

Waddington, I. (2019), Changing patterns of drug use in professional cycling: implications for anti doping policy, in B Fincoeur, J. Gleaves and F. Ohl (eds), Doping in Cycling, London, Routledge, 31–44.

Waddington, I. and Moller, V., (2019), WADA at twenty: old problems and old thinking?, *Internatioanl Journal of Sport Policy and Politics*, 11 (2), 203–218.

Waddington, I. and Smith, A. (2009), *An Introduction to Drugs in Sport: Addicted to Winning?* London, Routledge.

Wadler G. and Hainline, B . (1989), *Drugs and the Athlete*, Philadelphia, PA, F. A. Davis.
Weaver, S. (1985), Eyewitness: Tom Dickson, MD, describes procedures at the LA Olympics, *Bicycling* (Emmaus, Pa), March, 58–59.
Williams, J. G. P. and Sperryn, P. (eds) (1976), *Sports Medicine*, 2nd ed., London, Edward Arnold.
Williams, M. (1981), Blood doping: an update, *Physician and Sports Medicine*, 9, 59–64.
Williams, M., Lindhjem, M. and Schuster, R. (1978), The effect of blood infusion upon endurance capacity and ratings of perceived exertion, *Medicine and Science in Sports*, 10, 113–118.

Part 3

Sports medicine and drugs

The development of sports medicine in France

8 The medical embrace of sport in modern France

With Jeffrey Montez de Oca

In many western countries, and perhaps most notably in the UK and the United States, sports medicine after 1945 developed 'organically', that is as an aspect of the medical profession more generally, without significant external intervention or control by the central government. However, an important exception to this general western pattern was France, in which the state played a central role in the development of both sport and sports medicine (Brissonneau, 2003). Although the degree of centralised control was not as great as in the Soviet Union and East Germany, where sports medicine developed as an integral part of a state-sponsored and state-controlled sports system (Riordan, 1991; Spitzer, 2000, 2006; Dennis, 2015), the pattern of development in France was significantly different from that in most other western countries. For this reason, this section of the book focuses on a detailed case study which highlights some of the particular features of the development of sports medicine in France.

The central object of this chapter is to examine the central role of the state in France in the development of sports medicine after the Second World War, and the ways in which the state elevated the status of sports physicians to the role of key personnel in the search for improved sporting performances. In this regard it might be said that France represented a very different pattern of development of sports medicine in which the state was – in marked contrast to other western societies – a key actor in the medicalisation of sport. However, and notwithstanding the distinctive aspects of the pattern of French development, the outcome was very similar to that in other western societies: the extension of medical control into all aspects of sports training and competition at the elite level and the growing involvement of sports physicians in the search for enhanced performances.

In early twentieth-century France, the medical profession promoted some forms of physical activity but this did not normally include competitive sports. The general medical consensus in France at that time was that competitive physical activity pushed the body to and beyond harmful limits (Defrance, 1998). But in the early 1950s, some doctors began promoting sport for its claimed health benefits. In part, this change was associated with the fact that many of the younger doctors who promoted sport were themselves former sportspeople (Viaud, 2009) who were passionate supporters of competitive sports. In arguing the case for sport they were able to point to Hans Selye's (1946) concept of the General Adaptation Syndrome

DOI: 10.4324/9781003563921-12

(GAS), which turned the medical understanding of competitive sport on its head. Georges Pin (1951) explained in the pages of *Médecine, éducation physique et sport* that this new understanding of the GAS opened a new field of scientific research on the positive impact of exercise on the body since it provided a medical explanation for how physical stress causes positive reactions in the body that make it stronger (Pin, 1951). But of critical significance was the fact that the socio-economic-political situation of France in the immediate post-war period, on both the national and international levels, meant that key decision-makers, especially in the national government, were particularly receptive to the message of the enthusiastic physician-athletes in France.

Investing in a modern sport system

Ten years after the Second World War the effects of malnutrition were still visible in France. French agricultural production in the early post-war period was down 30 per cent compared to 1938. The war had ravaged the French economy and the post-war recovery was slow (Bossuat, 1986) and, as a result, a majority of the French population endured a meagre standard of living until the early 1960s. One of the numerous consequences of widespread malnutrition was the poor physical development of young people in France. Physicians alerted the Ministry of Health to the fact that France had experienced a decrease in the size of children and an increase in the number of skeletal disorders after 1945 (Berges, 1948).

Within this context, it was argued that physical education and diet were central to improving the health of young people, especially the development of their bones and skeletons, while the French government agreed that building healthy citizens and workers was necessary for recovery from the war. Jean Masson, State Secretary for Youth and Sports, argued that supervision of sport and physical activity should be handed over to medical professionals (Masson, 1952), a policy which greatly increased the remit of the medical profession by opening up new areas for medical practice and control. The medical profession was thus able to intervene in the curriculum of sport teachers by strongly influencing the *Instructions Officielles* (official programmes) for physical activities both in primary and secondary schools (Loudcher and Vivier, 1999). It also developed medical sport centres throughout France to provide medical care for young people. There were around one hundred sport medical centres in 1950 where physicians delivered annual sport certificates for club athletes after providing biometric screening (Encausse, 1951), for example monitoring different bodily functions. The medical centres also provided care for sports injuries of children as well as amateurs and elite sportspeople. The development of sport medical centres began slowly (115 in 1967) and then accelerated rapidly (185 by 1970) (Guillet and Génèty, 1975). Centres of expertise were created in Paris, Nancy and Bordeaux in the late 1950s for elite athletes. These centres were staffed by general practitioners who provided medical care for sportspeople and also carried out some scientific research. They also provided biometric screening and did some testing of athletes' physical capabilities such as flexibility, stamina and coordination.

However, the use of sport to strengthen the post-war nation did not end with the health of young people, for sport also came to be viewed by government as a means to increase France's international prestige. This involved the development of a highly centralised, state-sponsored system of sports medicine for elite athletes.

State-sponsored sports medicine and elite sport in France

Following the 1960 Olympics in Rome, the French team returned home without a single gold medal (Loret, 2008). The French media framed this as a national disgrace with important implications for the international status of France, since sport during the Cold War had increasingly become a political and cultural battleground between the capitalist 'Free World' and the communist system in Eastern Europe (Montez de Oca, 2013). The importance of international sporting events was ratcheted up because France at that time was seeking to increase its status as a world power. Following the Rome Olympics, President Charles de Gaulle decided that, within this context of changing international power dynamics, sport was too important to be left to the sport federations and that a centralised state policy was essential to develop sport (Fleuriel, 2004). He had already appointed Maurice Herzog, a world-renowned sportsman who was the first person to climb Annapurna in 1950, as High Commissioner for Sport in 1958. But France, it was held, also needed a national sport system (Lassus, Martin and Villaret, 2007). At this time, there were two dominant high-performance sport models, the liberal model in the United States and the centralised state model in the German Democratic Republic (GDR). The US system had relatively open training centres; athletes did not necessarily live on site and had regular interactions with outsiders. The GDR system was based on a closed system of sport centres that included on site everything needed for training, such as state-of-the-art equipment, coaches, doctors, restaurants and living quarters. Since these structures were closed, athletes rarely left and had limited interaction with outsiders. France adopted a model which had several features of the GDR model, which led to the centralisation and rationalisation of sport by the state (see Beamish and Ritchie, 2006: 85–104).

Under Herzog's direction, several steps were taken in order to professionalise sport. Firstly, the government imposed upon sports federations the need to renew the delegation of powers which they had been given by the state (decree of 27 November 1960). Since these delegated powers allowed federations to receive a state budget and to determine national champions, the requirement to renew their delegated power was an important lever of state control over the federations. And with the law of 6 August 1963, Herzog created a sports educator diploma to prepare coaches in scientific sport training, and these coaches were appointed to federal training centres at the national and regional levels. As a result, sports coaches in France were required to have a diploma in sport sciences delivered by the Sport Ministry.

Herzog's interventionist political strategy continued when Joseph Comiti succeeded him as Minister of Youth and Sport (1968–74). A higher-level state diploma of sport educator was created as a requirement for national coaches to work in a sport federation (decree of 15 June 1972). To encourage the development of more elite athletes nationally, *sections sport-études* were created as coach-managed sport centres within middle and high schools. Young athletes would study and train in these centres for five days a week (circulaire 74-136, 8 May 1974). The creation in 1975 of the National Institute for Sport and Physical Education (INSEP) represented another major step towards state centralisation. INSEP allowed elite athletes to study for a state diploma of sport educator in between their two training sessions per day, which facilitated their becoming state sport trainers upon retirement. From the 1960s until the 1990s, both coaching and the management of French federations were increasingly professionalised.

Alongside these changes in coaching and in the organisation of the sports federations, the French state also played a central role in the medicalisation of elite sport by creating medical structures within each national sports institution, so that elite sport and the provision of sports medicine in France became increasingly heavily directed by the state. In the following section we examine the importance of the development of this state-sponsored process of the medicalisation of sport in France in the middle years of the twentieth century.

The rise of sports medicine in the mid-twentieth century

The convergence of domestic politics (national health concerns) and international politics (France's position within the global order) combined to promote the importance of sports medicine in the 1950s, 1960s and 1970s. As we have noted, the state invested resources into sports medicine and medical infrastructure across the country. Sports doctors enjoyed increased access to the population, one key aspect of which was that sports doctors gained increased control over the development and supervision of sports training for everyone from schoolchildren to elite athletes.

Central to the mission of sports doctors was the professionalisation of sport by supervising the training of physical educators and sports coaches. This meant that training was to be guided by scientific analysis, rationality and efficiency rather than 'empiricism' (training according to traditional knowledge and bodily sensations).[1] Herzog underlined the role of the medical profession in a symposium on Sport and Medicine: 'As I have said many times, we have left the time of empiricism. We have a duty to seek the invaluable contribution of scholars, and to draw the broadest benefit' (Herzog, 1965: 9–11). Professor Albert Govaerts, President of the International Federation of Sports Medicine, set out his view of the goal of sports medicine in his closing statement to the 10th International Congress of Sports Medicine in 1954:

> sports medicine has a specifically defined purpose: studying a human being who is capable within a few seconds of moving from a system capacity of approximately ¼ HP in the resting state to 12 HP … for long distance races. What are those mechanisms? What are the limits of this extraordinary power?
>
> (Govaerts, 1954: 23)

The mission of sports medicine according to Govaerts is to study human physical potential and its limits. As we shall see in the next chapter, fatigue sets a natural limit on the human body's physical capabilities and, therefore, defines the limits of human potential. As sports medicine continued to become increasingly integrated with elite sport, its goal was to constantly extend the horizon of human potential. It pursued that goal by developing technologically sophisticated training regimes which, as we shall see in the next chapter, included pharmaceutical support. In the next section, we outline how sports medicine became increasingly integrated with elite sport.

Sports medicine and the medicalisation of elite sport

According to a 1962 press release published in *L'Equipe* (July 9) by Dr Pierre Dumas, official physician of the Tour de France, 12 riders had become sick and dropped out of the race before the start of the stage from Luchon. The riders claimed their sudden indisposition was caused by the fish they had eaten the previous night. Dr Dumas rejected their claim since most of the sick riders were on the same team while riders on other teams were not sick. Moreover, the riders with the worst gastric disorders had not eaten the fish. Dumas concluded that the riders had become sick as a result of poorly administered drug cocktails (*L'Equipe*, July 9, 1962). Since 1952, when he first became the official physician of the Tour de France, Dr Dumas had seen and condemned drug use by riders. His primary concern was the non-scientific way in which soigneurs (former cyclists who provide a range of different types of personal care to riders) provided medical treatment that was 'empirical', that is based on folk knowledge, personal experience and intuition. (It might be noted that in England, doctors involved in the treatment of athletes similarly deplored what they regarded as the 'backwards', or 'superstitious' or 'faddy' habits of non-medically qualified coaches or trainers. See Heggie, 2011: 70.) Dumas also saw that the riders were willing to take whatever their soigneurs recommended in order to gain a competitive advantage (Marchand, 1959: 4).

The story of the fish is typically understood as the incident that motivated Dumas to organise, in the following year, the First European Conference on Doping in Uriage-les-Bains that, in turn, produced France's first formal anti-doping law. However, the anecdote illustrates something else as well. Dumas was a man of science but he had also been a successful athlete himself – he held a black belt in judo – and so was already a partial insider to the world of elite sport before becoming the doctor to the Tour de France. When he gained access to elite cycling, he was horrified by the unprofessional, non-scientific care that sportspeople received. He saw the riders' treatments as informed by myth and mysticism rather than medical science. Treatment by soigneurs, Dumas believed, would lead to more tragedies and scandals, such as when Jean Mallejac collapsed on Mont Ventoux during the 1955 Tour de France (Mignon, 2003: 231). The logical conclusion for Dumas was to minimise the role of amateurs who could do harm and to put professional physicians in charge of supervising the training and care of elite sportspeople. Doing so would increase the application of medical science and decrease the application of what he considered to be dangerous empiricism.

Rationalising the national sport system

The movement towards the medicalisation of elite sports training can be seen in the rationalisation of sport training centres by physicians. The National Institute of Sport (INS), created in 1945 and located in Bois de Vincennes, near Paris, had been established to implement a national sports policy and to provide the best training facilities for French champions. From our current vantage point, the organisation of INS in the 1950s through the early 1970s may seem quite casual. Not all of the athletes lived at the Institute. Some stayed in their local region. Sport was not their primary occupation; it was a passion that they pursued in addition to their primary job, while medical support at INS was provided by doctors who were general practitioners rather than doctors with specialist sports-related knowledge. The doctors would be available to meet athletes at INS and also travelled with the athletes to national and international competitions. However, and most importantly, consultations between athletes and doctors normally took place only *after an injury had occurred*. Thus interactions between athletes and doctors tended to focus solely on the treatment of injuries while the non-specialist general practitioners also used older, traditional, methods for treating injuries, such as applying a bloody beef steak to contusions.

Leading sports doctors in the 1950s and 1960s argued that amateurism in the French sport system was holding France back in international competition. They also argued that elite athletes could benefit from their more specialised and advanced skills. In the opening speech of the 12th Congress of the International Federation of Sports Medicine, Professor Albert Govaerts envisioned increasing the role of physicians in the training regimes of elite athletes:

> The formula for maximum performance stands at present: sportsperson + coach + sports doctor + comprehensive employer. The performance might be even better with the following formula: sportsperson + *coaching physician* + comprehensive employer.
>
> (Govaerts, 1958: 19–20, emphasis added)

In 1950, Dr Alain Richard, professor at the University of Paris and former president of the French Medical Society of Physical Education and Sport, argued that doctors were key to developing sporting performance by providing medical supervision to training. Doctors' scientific knowledge helps them 'to identify some pathophysiological trends that impeded the progress of sporting effort' (Richard, 1950: 111). Sports medicine, he argued, was able to calculate the necessary changes in dosage of pharmaceuticals and even 'to correct them clinically' (Richard, 1950: 111).

Adopting the state-centred East German sport system facilitated the movement from the casual organisation of sport centres staffed by general practitioners to highly rationalised centres where exercise physiologists developed specialised training regimes for athletes to follow *before they were injured*. We can see here very clearly the process of the medicalisation of sport, in which the role of doctors changes from a marginal role, simply treating the injuries of athletes, to a much more central role in the planning, preparation and everyday supervision of athletes' training regimes with a view to enhancing performance.

The first step towards this new elite state sports structure was the creation in 1967 of a high altitude 'sports high school' in Font Romeu, in the Pyrenees.[2] Modelled on the closed sports centres in the GDR, the buildings were laid out in a small village and cut off from the outside world. As with all aspects of the school, the built environment was designed to focus on the training and performance of talented young athletes. Athletes had at their disposal a restaurant, living quarters, and the best sports facilities and coaches. The campus had a state-of-the-art medical centre to treat injuries and a medical research centre to improve performance. Athletes from many different nations and many different sports attended Font Romeu to enjoy the positive effects altitude has on 'health'. All of the athletes came together in the cafeteria to eat, drink, joke and commiserate about the rigours of training. Athletes would also discuss among themselves issues relating to health, training methods, recovery, doctors and 'recovery means', over coffee or beer.

In the 1970s, a national network of specialist sports studies sections was created in high schools to provide specialist coaching and facilities for the most talented young athletes. Class schedules were changed to allow for intensive daily training sessions and medical performance monitoring. In 1974 there were 55 sport studies sections with 1180 students and by 1982 this had increased to 181 sections with 4044 students. Students who did not live near a section could stay in a boarding school. They took classes together and trained five times a week and took part in competitions or training camps at the weekends. These elite training centres were linked to nearby hospitals that engaged in medical research on human physical performance and the young athletes regularly went to these research centres where doctors tested their cardiovascular system and their blood to provide guidance on the quality of their training.

The political will to professionalise the National Institute of Sport (INS) came after France's disappointing results at the 1972 Munich Olympics. In 1975, under the direction of Pierre Mazeaud, Secretary of State for Youth, Sports and Recreation, a high-level, state-of-the-art training centre was established. This involved the merger of the INS and the Normal School of Physical Education (ENSEP), which had produced the best physical education teachers, to form the National Institute of Sport and Physical Education (INSEP), also known as the National Sport Centre. This was the beginning of the truly modern era in elite French sport. At INSEP, athletes could train in state-of-the-art facilities with certified national coaches working in close association with the best sports doctors. In 1977, an Olympics Preparation Mission was drafted to define the objectives for both individual and collective training programmes. It further ensured that the best athletes had enough financial support to offset the costs of high-level training. And finally, the new system centrally regulated the heterodox array of federal sport policies.

The increasing importance of sports doctors and sports medicine

Following the GDR model, the French state created a system in which sports doctors were increasingly given responsibility for supervising high-level athletes, with training regimes based on modern science rather than on traditional, empirical knowledge. In 1968, Herzog developed a medical department in the Ministry of Youth and Sport. With Law n° 75988, Pierre Mazeaud, who was one of Herzog's successors, integrated a medical commission into each sports federation in order to guarantee their efficiency and to promote the 'health' of athletes. Henri Théret, Deputy to the State Secretary of Sports and Youth, stated, '[The medical profession] must develop the knowledge to monitor high-level competitive sportspeople who are involved in the search for higher and higher records and performance' (Théret, 1967: 7). Dr Jacques Pruvost was a physician at the National Institute of Sport in the 1970s when it became INSEP. In an interview with Brissonneau (October 3, 2002), he described the professionalisation of medicine at INSEP when general practitioners gave way to research physicians:

> What was important in high performance sport was micro-traumatology. That is a little something that prevents the elite athlete from obtaining the last hundredth of a second. These are notions that can be acquired through experience. We must follow the athlete for years to get to know their habits, their sleep, their way of life. Anything can be an influence, even small things. It takes almost one doctor to one elite athlete.

A key development which further entrenched the central role of physicians in elite level sport was the establishment of a network of Regional Institutes of Sports Medicine, of which there were 18 by 1975. The establishment of this network of regional institutes was an important development because of their close integration with local university hospital centres, which allowed for the systematic medical monitoring of training, the development of sports traumatology techniques, the teaching of sports biology and scientific research in a university and hospital network. The significance of this development in the medicalisation of sport in France has been precisely recognised by Viaud, who describes it as 'without doubt the most remarkable advance in sports medicine in the 1970s: *physical activity and athletes entered the hospital*' ('c'est là sans aucun doute l'avancée la plus remarquable de la décennie soixante-dix en matière de médecine du sport: les activités physiques et les athlètes font leur entrée à l'hopital' [Viaud, 2009: 344, emphasis added]).

To help athletes improve their performances, doctors, especially researchers in the field of exercise physiology, sought more control to supervise sports training to generate greater sporting success for France. The problem, as the doctors saw it, was that coaches were guided by empiricism rather than science. Professor Chailley-Bert, the first holder of a chair in sports medicine, held that inadequate preparation and a lack of physicians explained the poor performance of French athletes at the 1960 Winter Games in Squaw Valley. He argued that while a tremendous amount of money had been invested in French preparation for the Olympics, the nation was not seeing a proper return on this investment. 'In an international competition in which the cost is so high, whose results have an impact on the standing of our country, is it right, is it reasonable, to give the responsibility of the national team only to coaches … without the assistance of a competent physician' (Chailley-Bert, 1959: 151).[3] While recognising the coaches' talent, he also saw them as amateurs lacking in scientific knowledge. Chailley-Bert believed doctors should take on the role of lead trainers so that they could study the athletes to generate usable scientific knowledge about human performance and potential.

Researchers such as Chailley-Bert were similarly dissatisfied with the education and training that physical and sports education teachers were receiving in universities and clubs. In 1964, after returning from the convention of FIMS and the International Federation of Physical Education (IFPE) in Tokyo, he argued that physical education and sports education teachers were presenting reports that were not based on up-to-date knowledge. He further criticised them for not implementing power training which, he held, put France at a significant competitive disadvantage (Chailley-Bert, 1966).

In 1959 and in 1966, Chailley-Bert argued that doctors should be able to intervene in the 'care' of elite athletes. He stated that, if the Czech runner Emil Zátopek had won three gold medals at Helsinki in 1952, it was because doctors had 'remade' him (Chailley-Bert, 1966: 99). It was argued that sports physicians had the specialised scientific knowledge and skills to carry out physiological tests on athletes and advise coaches on exactly when to moderate or intensify the training programme. As we noted earlier, this represented an important extension of medical control within sport; no longer was the doctor's role confined to the treatment, or even the prevention, of injuries, for the doctors' scientific knowledge was becoming increasingly central in pushing athletes to their physical and mental limits in the search for enhanced performance. Dr Pierre-Henri Périé, a physician working for the Secretariat of the Ministry of Youth and Sports, agreed and delineated four sub-specialities of sports medicine in training top sportspeople (1971: 11–12):

1. Preventive medicine: this should determine an athlete's ability to engage in physical activity and when to rest. It advises on the most relevant activities for an athlete according to their physical condition. It should also teach health monitoring to future physical education and sports teachers so that teachers can be preventative actors in the development of young people.
2. Medical care and traumatology: an area of sports medicine focused on treating sports injuries, with a clear recognition of the need for doctors to quickly 'repair' injuries so that athletes can return to training and competition as quickly as a possible.
3. Medical monitoring of high-performance training: the doctor advises coaches and gives them 'objective' data for the selection of sportspeople for competitions. As Périé stated, 'the coach needs (1971, 11) to have precise physiological information with regards to individual possibilities'. These doctors can interpret data at an emotional, sensory-motor, and physiological level, which is beyond the skill of coaches. They also help to develop the most effective

overload training, i.e. the gradual increase of stress placed upon the body to develop strength and power.

4. Medical research applied to sport: research studies based on elite sportspeople can generate useful knowledge about human limits, especially in relation to the impact of fatigue.

Périé argued that previously medicine had been largely limited to studying sick patients. Elite-level competition provided the possibility of studying healthy humans in motion rather than resting humans as had been done in most medical research (Périé, 1976: 55). Physical and sports activities also offered therapeutic possibilities in the treatment of many organic and mental health problems. Thus, the acquisition of data of this kind would help to develop collections of reference data (anthropometric and physiological) that could define what it means to be healthy and shed light on different physiological stages of intensive training. In sum, Périé wanted high-performance sport to become an applied research laboratory, with elite sportspeople as high-powered guinea pigs.

It will be recalled (in Chapter 3) that Heggie (2011: 30), in her history of sports medicine in Britain, had described three dimensions of sports medicine: (i) treatment; (ii) enhancement; and (iii) prevention and that she argued that in Britain in the first few decades of the twentieth century, while basic treatment of injuries certainly occurred there was little evidence of either enhancement or prevention. It will also be recalled that Cronin (2007: 265–27) has similarly noted that even those doctors with an interest in sport at this time 'were not overly concerned ... with offering sports medicine to sportsmen as something that could be consumed as a way of improving their performance, or ensuring they return to full fitness in as quick a time as possible'. Périé's characterisation of the many aspects of sports medicine indicates how strikingly the remit of sports medicine had expanded beyond simply the provision of medical care for injuries and, we might add, how this most basic aspect of sports medicine was already becoming increasingly subject to the constraint to get 'players fit yesterday' (Waddington et. al, 1999: 26) in order to return athletes to training and competition as quickly as possible.

Within this expanded role for sports physicians, the idea that sports medicine should participate in the development of sports performance became central to its mission. Dr Andrivet, a traumatologist and the medical director of the National Institute of Sport, argued that sports medicine is 'medical care that allows for quickly treating normal or sports injuries that disrupt training' (Andrivet, 1971: 23). Dr Catherine Defoligny, who succeeded Dr Périé as medical chief of staff of the Ministry of Youth and Sports, added that sports medicine provides both diagnostic care and preventative care, i.e. medical screening, developing training regimes and helping to understand the impacts of intensive training (Defoligny, 1981: 30). By the 1970s and 1980s, sports medicine had become an essential adjunct to elite sports training and performance.

Conclusion

In France, as in the UK, one can see in the period after 1945 the steady expansion of the role of sports physicians in the training and preparation of athletes, and especially of elite athletes. In France, this was part of a deliberate strategy to improve the performance of French athletes in international competition and the key difference between France and the UK was that, in France, this process of the medicalisation of sport was largely sponsored by, and supported by, the French government whereas in the UK it was a development which was led by the profession itself – or at least by that section of the profession who were interested and involved in the care, treatment and preparation of athletes. But in France, too, the extension of medical authority into sport was enthusiastically supported by sports physicians, their central argument being the need for training programmes to be based on science rather than traditional, 'empirical' practices, and that only they had the medical and scientific expertise to determine the appropriate training schedules and routines for athletes, and their preparation before international competitions.

In the next chapter, we examine how this increasingly central role of sports medicine in elite sport and in the search for enhanced performances led French sports physicians to recommend the use of pharmacological products.

Notes

1 The terms 'empirical' and 'empiricism' carry particular connotations in French sports sciences. In French sport sciences, they are pejorative terms used to connote subjective, experiential-based knowledge that lacks scientific rigour or theorisation. Empiricism in sport training is seen as anachronistic and in need of being replaced by science. See Beaudou, A. 2001. Science et empirisme en éducation physique, in Saint-Martin, J.-P. (ed.) *Histoire d'EPS*. Paris: Vigot.

2 The information in this section is based on conversations between Brissonneau and Pierre Mazeaud and national trainers at the symposium 'La loi Mazeaud du 29 octobre 1975 relative au développement de l'éducation physique et du sport: Loi de synthèse ou affirmation de l'Etat?' June 13, 2006.

3 Although the Squaw Valley Games were held in 1960, the publication date of this issue of *Médecine, Education Physique et Sport* was 1959. We suspect this had to do with the publication's limited operating budget.

References

Andrivet, R. (1971), Les rapports de la médecine du sport et de l'entraînement, *Médecine du sport*, 1, 23–24.

Beamish, R. and Ritchie, I. (2006), *Fastest, Highest, Strongest. A Critique of High-Performance Sport*, London, Routledge.

Berges, H. (1948), Répercussions des calamités de guerre sur la première enfance, *Population*, 3, 501–518.

Bossuat, G. (1986), L'aide américaine à la France après la seconde guerre mondiale, *Vingtième Siècle*, revue d'histoire, 9, 17–36.

Brissonneau, C. (2003), *Entrepreneurs de morale et carrières de deviants dans le dopage sportif: prises de position er témoignages vécus dans la médecine du sport et dans deux disciplines sportives, l'athlétisme et le cyclisme sur la route (1960–2002)*, PhD dissertation, Paris X Nanterre University.

Chailley-Bert, P. (1959), Conclusions, *Médecine, éducation physique et sport*, 3, 151–153.
Chailley-Bert, P. (1966), L'orientation moderne de la médecine du sport, *Médecine du sport*, 1, 97–101.
Cronin, M, (2007), Not taking the medicine: sportsmen and doctors in late nineteenth-century Britain, *Journal of Sport History*, 34 (1), 23–35.
Defoligny, C. (1981), Où en est la médecine du sport en France, *Médecine du sport*, 55 (5), 4–5.
Defrance, J. (1998), Sport, santé et institution médicale, *Prévenir*, 34 (1), 85–91.
Dennis, M. (2015), The East German doping programme, in V. Møller, I. Waddington and J. Hoberman (eds), *Routledge Handbook of Drugs and Sport*, Routledge, Abingdon, 170–180.
Encausse, P. (1951), *Sport et santé,* Paris, Amédée Legrand.
Fleuriel, S. (2004), *Le sport de haut niveau en France. Sociologie d'une catégorie de pensée,* Grenoble, Presses universitaires de Grenoble.
Govaerts, A. (1954), Rapport du 10ème congrès international de médecine sportive, 10ème Congrès International de Médecine Sportive, Belgrade, 23–24.
Govaerts, A. (1958), Rapport du 12ème congrès international de médecine sportive, 12ème Congrès International de Médecine Sportive, Moscow, 15–20.
Guillet, R. and Génety, J. (1975), *Abrégé de médecine du sport,* Paris, Masson.
Heggie, V. (2011), *A History of British Sports Medicine*, Manchester, Manchester University Press.
Herzog, M. (1965), Allocutions. *Compte rendu du colloque international Sport et Médicine: Vichy 1964*, Paris: Ed. L. R. d'Art.
Lassus, M., Martin, J. L. and Villaret, S. (2007), Les politiques publiques du sport (1945 à nos jours), in P. Têtart (ed.), *Histoire du sport. De la Libération à nos jours*, Paris, Vuibert.
Loret, A. (2008), *Le sport de la république. La France face au défi Olympique*, Paris, Du Temps.
Loudcher, J. and Vivier, C. (1999), La santé dans l'histoire de l'éducation physique. Analyse des conceptions de la normalité à travers la méthode de Pierre Seurin, in J. Gleyse (ed.), *Approches historique et culturelle*, Paris, Vigot, 81–97.
Marchand, J. (1959), Nouvelle alerte au doping, *L'Equipe*, 4, 14 July.
Masson, J. (1952), Allocution. IX Congrès International de Médecine Sportive, Paris, 13–17.
Mignon, P. (2003), The Tour de France and the doping issue, in H. Dauncy and G. Hare (eds.), *The Tour de France 1903–2003*, London, Cass, 227–245.
Montez De Oca, J. (2013), *Discipline and Indulgence: College Football, Media, and the American Way of Life During the Cold War,* New Brunswick, NJ: Rutgers University Press.
Perie. P.-H. (1971), Options actuelles de la médicine du sport. Multiplications des problèmes de santé en relation avec les transformations de l'environnement. *Médecine du sport,* 1, 7–15.
Périé, P.-H. (1976), Coordination des actions de recherche. Actualité d'un conseil supérieur de la medécine du sport, *Médecine du sport*, 50, 54–58.
Pin, G. (1951), Les possibilités d'application du 'syndrome général d'adaptation' au contrôle médical des sports, *Médecine, éducation physique et sport*, 1, 7–32.
Richard, A. (1950), La surveillance médicale de l'entraînement aux exercices de fond, *Médecine, education physique et sport*, 3, 111–122.
Riordan, J. (1991), *Sport. Politicsi and Communism,* Manchester, Manchester University Press.
Selye, H. (1946), The general adaptation syndrome and the diseases of adaptation, *Journal of Allergy and Clinical Immunology*, 17, 231–247.
Spitzer, G. (2000), *Doping in der DDR*, Köln, Bundesinstitut für Sportwissenschaft.

Spitzer, G. (2002), Ranking number 3 in the world: How the addiction to doping changed sport in the GDR, in G. Spitzer (ed). *Doping and Doping Control in Euroope*, Oxford, Meyer and Meyer, 57–77.

Théret, H. (1967), Allocution de monsieur Henri Théret, *Médecine, education physique et sport*, 1, 7.

Viaud, B. (2009), *Panser les deux mondes. Médecines et sports, entre principes hippocratiques et performances*, PhD Dissertation, Université de Nantes.

Waddington, I., Roderick, M. and Parker, G. (1999), *Managing Injuries in Professional Football: A Study of the Roles of the Club Doctor and Physiotherapist*, Leicester, Centre for Research into Sport and Society, University of Leicester.

9 The structural ambivalence of sports medicine

With Jeffrey Montez de Oca

The central object of this chapter is to analyse how the increasing involvement of physicians in elite sport created a series of ironies and contradictions. As we shall see, sports doctors in France introduced scientific training methods in order to help French athletes compete more effectively in international competitions. Those methods led to more intensive training which placed far greater demands on the bodies of athletes. And while these methods were aimed at improving performances, a further consequence of more intensive scientific training was that athletes sustained more injuries and experienced greater fatigue (Brissonneau, 2003; Le Breton, 2010: 158; Rouanet, 2014: 135). To treat their patients and prepare them for forthcoming international competitions, sports doctors provided athletes with more and more medications to protect their health. This produced a fairly simple equation: more intensive training caused athletes to experience more fatigue which in turn created the need for more recovery time. In order to reduce recovery time and keep French athletes competitive, French sports doctors followed the pharmacological strategies of doctors in other top sporting nations. The scientisation of sport and the increased fatigue that it created thus led to the increased use of pharmacology among elite international athletes, a process which was first called 'biological preparation' and, later, 'hormonal rebalancing' (Bellocq and Bressan, 1991). The commitment to international sporting success spurred the growth of sports medicine and, at the same time, made sports doctors ever more central players in elite sport. A result of the contradictions within elite sport at this time was to blur the line between those pharmaceutical products which were prescribed to enhance athletic performance (and which were labelled as doping) and the prescription of those pharmacological products which were deemed necessary to protect the athletes' health (and considered as a part of healthcare provision).

An important aspect of this story is the competing roles taken by different doctors. Some doctors acted as trainers and healers for athletes while others acted as anti-doping moral entrepreneurs, policing athletes and their trainers. Physicians' differing positions on doping were largely determined by their work situation, that is by their professional location in the medical field and their relationships to sportspeople. Doctors who made a living preparing athletes for international competitions and those who made a living policing the behaviours of sportspeople tended to define doping differently (Brissonneau, 2003). This not only led to debates about

DOI: 10.4324/9781003563921-13

the meaning of doping (what is considered health promoting versus what is considered as cheating) and to different approaches to anti-doping policies and programmes, but it also led to the involvement of sports physicians in repeated doping scandals and crises in elite sport.

Fatigue: crossing the chemical barrier to performance enhancement

If we wish to understand the relationship between sports medicine and doping it is important to understand that the everyday work situations of sports physicians are structurally ambivalent. Doctors' differing professional positions in elite sport create conflicting interests, motivations and attitudes towards pharmacology. This structural ambivalence has been associated with the instrumental role of some doctors in the proliferation of the use of pharmacology in elite sport. In this section, we address the structural situation of sports physicians which leads some doctors – notwithstanding their commitment to codes of medical ethics – to prescribe banned drugs. In order to understand this, it is important to recognise that this cannot be understood simply as a question of deviant motivation on an individual, psychological level; rather, it has to be understood in terms of the structural organisation of elite sport itself and the increasingly central role of sports physicians within elite sport.

One of the major barriers that elite sportspeople and their trainers face during training and in competitions is fatigue. Fatigue is a natural barrier that protects the body from the dangers of overexertion. Crossing that natural barrier may be dangerous. While a win-at-all-costs attitude in competition demands pushing all the boundaries, Professor Lemarchands warned at the first international symposium on doping, held at Uriage-les-Bains in 1963, that it could be harmful:

> It [fatigue] announces the time when the maximum human ability is reached and no more can be asked of the body without seriously compromising its balance ... To want to remove this sign is to ignore the defences that the body puts in place to maintain its biological characteristics.
>
> (Lemarchands, 1964: 23)

In the middle years of the twentieth century, amphetamines were the most widely used drugs by sportspeople, especially cyclists, because they helped athletes ignore the signs of fatigue and avoid the decline in performance associated with fatigue. However, Professor Giuseppe La Cava (who later became president of FIMS in 1968) suggested that the use of amphetamines could be dangerous:

> They remove warning signs... [such as] the sensations of fatigue (i.e. the alarm by which nature tells us that our bodies cannot exceed this limit without serious danger) but they do not eliminate the fatigue itself and the toxins it produces.
>
> (La Cava, 1954: 25)

The Italian delegation to the meeting of the Extra-School Committee of the Council of Europe in January 1963 agreed that stimulants suppressed the warning signs of fatigue that kept people from exceeding their physiological frontiers. Dr Pierre Bugard (deputy head of the laboratory of endocrinology at the Parisian hospital Laennec) argued that 'anti-fatigue medication should not seek to hide tiredness but to slow down catabolism and promote anabolism and restoration'. To achieve that end, he suggested giving athletes not only vitamins and minerals, but also hormones (cited in Guillet, 1964: 71).

The views of doctors who opposed doping because of what was seen as its artificial, i.e. non-natural, character, also tended to be ambivalent and self-contradictory. For instance, Dr Guy Duchesnay suggested that doctors intervene before the onset of fatigue by administering molecules of substances such as amphetamines, strychnine or caffeine (Duchesnay, 1959: 293). However, those products do not occur naturally in the body but must be artificially added. The recommendations by doctors such as Duchesnay thus offered technological solutions developed through pharmacological techniques (*les techniques biologiques*) that ignored the 'artificial' aspect of their endeavour. And in asserting the technical solutions to these problems, they were of course also asserting the central role of sports doctors in the training process. Duchesnay recognised that above a certain quantity, the drugs he recommended to delay fatigue were dangerous, and therefore it was the role of the physician to prescribe the proper quantities of drugs for sportspeople to increase performance in a safe manner. In this regard it might be said that doctors were increasingly coming to see themselves not just as handmaidens to sports training but, rather, as the overseers.

The view of the medical office of the Youth and Sports Ministry was that the medical profession should manage 'the fight against fatigue under strict medical monitoring' (Crespin, 1968: 25). The critical phrase here was, of course, 'under medical monitoring', since it recognised the central controlling role of the doctor in the preparation of athletes. In other words, doctors should monitor all aspects of the training process to protect the health of elite athletes and to ensure the best preparation for international competition. Medical monitoring by the medical profession, it was assumed, could resolve the tension between caring for the athletes' health and enhancing their ability to win medals in international competitions. The French state, in the form of the Youth and Sports Ministry, had effectively given its formal approval to the central role of sports physicians in preparing French athletes for competition.

Doctors were thus invested with great power to redesign the French sports system and they did so from the perspective of medical professionals who were deeply involved in and committed not just to the world of medicine, but also to the world of sport and to the key goal of sporting success. As medical professionals, it was simply logical to draw on scientific knowledge and apply medical technologies to solve problems within sport. However, by doing so they deepened the already existing contradictions and further extended the growing reach of doctors and medicine into the world of sports, a world which itself was already politically charged and which was about to become revolutionised by growing commercialisation and the development of global audiences, both of which would have the effect of placing even greater stress on the importance of winning.

The doctor-patient relationship in elite sport

In elite sport, sports doctors work closely with elite athletes, sometimes over prolonged periods of time. As a result, they see the athletes' pains and they know their dreams. No doubt most sports doctors seek to use their specialist knowledge and skills to help their athlete-patients to achieve their goals. However, many of the doctors' choices are complicated and ethically fraught because of their simultaneous commitment to what Coakley (2009: 163–166) has called the sport ethic – a key part of which is the commitment to sporting success – and their commitment to codes of medical ethics. Codes of medical ethics require that doctors must protect the health of their patients. However, in the world of elite sport, the concept of good health relates not merely to the absence of illness but to the athlete's ability to compete most effectively at full physical potential. Drawing upon their expertise to resolve that contradiction, many doctors from the 1960s advocated the use of pharmacology in ways that would now be labelled doping.

What underpinned doctors' support for the use of pharmacology was the claim that doctors alone have the knowledge and therefore the right to make judgements about the health of athletes. This gave doctors working with athletes the right – indeed, the obligation – to make medical interventions in athletes' training regimes to protect their health. For example, Dr René Guillet (doctor to the French Olympic Team in 1964, and president of the Lyonnaise region of the French Medical Society of Physical Education and Sport) argued:

> If, prior to a competition, the doctor attached to a sportsperson believes that a sportsperson's condition requires taking a drug which is regarded as doping, nothing prevents the doctor legally from prescribing the drug if he thinks it is appropriate for the state of the sportsperson at that time … Nothing forbids a doctor from 'treating' a sportsperson and prescribing, if it seems medically appropriate, amphetamines, steroids or painkillers.
>
> (Guillet, 1964: 13)

Guillet approvingly cited Professor André Cier (pharmacologist, and chef de la Division de Chimie et de Pharmacologie au Centre de Recherches du Service de Santé des Armées), for whom rationally treating fatigue should have the purpose of restoring or maintaining the physiological balance disrupted by intensive exercise. Guillet added that 'From a strictly pharmacological and medical point of view, to condemn a drug regardless of the doses at which it is administered seems absurd' (Guillet, 1964: 82). Cier argued that doctors' specialised medical knowledge allowed them alone to determine what is best for the physical and mental health of athletes and for their ability to compete at the highest level.

The claim to specialist medical and scientific knowledge underpinned the claim that doctors alone could determine what is healthy in relation to the care of athletes. In October 1967, in an open letter published in the cycling magazine *Miroir du cyclisme*, Dr Burger, a former deputy chief of the medical school of Strasbourg, drew a distinction between the prescription to cyclists of drugs for therapy and the prescription of (sometimes the same) drugs for doping. He argued that, in major stage races such as the Tour de France, cyclists could suffer temporary impairments to internal organs. In this case, taking a stimulant within the race was a form of therapy, rather than a form of doping, and he recommended the use of amphetamines as a therapeutic measure. Similarly, Dr Philippe Miserez, who was the doctor of the Tour de France in 1976, suggested in *Sports Magazine* that authorising the use of amphetamines was the lesser of two evils – the other 'evil' being the risk of damage to the body of the athlete by the intense level of competition – and was acceptable when it does not exceed a certain threshold (Miserez, 1976). It was up to the doctor, drawing on their expert medical knowledge, to prescribe acceptable dosages of these drugs to protect the health of riders. While many doctors did not agree with prescribing amphetamines to athletes there was growing agreement that only doctors, as opposed to people without medical qualifications, such as soigneurs, should monitor and treat cyclists. Holding up the French ski team as a successful model, Burger (1967) argued that doctors should apply scientific knowledge to the riders' dietetics, training, and 'biological preparation'.

The ambiguity of 'biological preparation'

'Biological preparation' was the phrase used to describe the action of doctors in prescribing medication to elite athletes to help them manage fatigue and speed up recovery during training. It is significant that this precise phrase was included in the title of the 1963 conference at Uriage-les-Bains: the European Conference on Doping and Biological Preparation of the Competitive Athlete. While there is no clear documentation on which specific substances were used for 'biological preparation', they probably included not just vitamins but also anabolic steroids (Ballester, 2015). For some French doctors, the definition of doping primarily located the use of drugs in competition, while 'biological preparation' referred to drugs prescribed days or weeks before an event to help sportspeople recover during training. Thus the difference between doping and biological preparation was temporal: doping referred to substances used for immediate results in competition while biological preparation was future oriented and referred to substances prescribed by a physician as an aid to training. Despite only minor differences, only one set of practices was stigmatised as doping.

The temporal differentiation between biological preparation and doping was held to be critical. Jacques-Robert Boissier, a professor of pharmacology, explained that products taken during or immediately before a competition were doping while those taken during training could be considered 'almost as part of a best and more balanced diet' (Boissier, 1964: 20). Dr Delezenne, a member of the Central Medical Board of the French Football Federation, said he opposed doping but endorsed 'biological preparation' that acted upon cellular metabolism, the transformation of foods, sugars, amino acids and some vitamins into energy. As a result, he advocated medical treatments that would help tired athletes to return quickly to their normal physical condition (Delezenne, 1963). The historian, trainer and athlete Johannès Pallierre saw biological preparation, or what he called 'means of support', as acceptable because it was used in preparation for, rather than in, competition. For Pallierre, the support which doctors provided to athletes during training helped them to achieve peak condition more quickly and more safely and to ensure better performances (Palliere, 1964: 40). It might be noted that, as we saw in Chapter 7, Pallierre used exactly the same term – 'means of support' – as the physicians in the state-sponsored doping programme in East Germany in the 1970s.

The report from the Commission of Athletes at the conference at Uriage les Bains, which was guided by physicians, offered the following definition of biological preparation:

> Biological preparation is a set of hygienic conditions, which are offered to athletes to improve their health and, consequently, their performance. This preparation is for personal hygiene, the constant monitoring of all training, i.e. looking for the best physical performance and psychological endurance, to the diet, with potential therapeutic or dietary supplements included in a medically controlled preparation: some vitamins, relaxation, etc ... Biological preparation must be supervised by a physician in conjunction with the manager and coach in a climate of mutual trust and respectful sportsmanship.
>
> (*Rapport de la Commission des Athlètes*, 1964: 52)

This definition highlighted the central role of doctors in managing the 'biology' of performance. And as practitioners of sports medicine attempted to push back against the natural phenomenon of fatigue, so they were also pushing at the boundaries of what might be considered legitimate medical intervention and what might be considered doping. The challenge was thus to know where 'biological preparation' ended and doping began, and only medical professionals, it was argued, could define that boundary. But the activities of sports physicians were making this boundary ever more blurred as, for example, when the medical office of the Youth and Sports Ministry, which was formally opposed to doping, asked doctors to 'take into account the exceptional performance' of professionals and 'allow for ... the struggle against fatigue under strict medical surveillance'.

Within this context it is important to bear in mind a point of fundamental importance: the concept of what constitutes doping is a value-laden concept which is socially generated by specific groups within specific socio-economic-political situations. The concept of doping is socially defined and has no inherent, unchanging or essential meaning. Instead, it takes on the meaning given to it by specific social groups at any given time and place. In other words, there is no procedure, technique or drug that can inherently or essentially be considered doping outside the social and political context within which that social judgement is made. Biological preparation in the 1960s involved medical interventions in training and the prescription of drugs to improve performance, but doctors involved in this process did not generally consider that it constituted doping, or that they were in any way acting improperly. As we move from the 1960s into the 1970s, and especially into more recent times, this dividing line became even more complex. The boundary between what were considered doctors' reasonable pharmacological interventions in elite sport training and what was considered doping shifted with the movement away from the term 'biological preparation' and the adoption of a new term: 'hormonal rebalancing'. In the rest of the chapter we look at the emergence of hormonal rebalancing and how different doctors involved in elite sport positioned themselves along the boundary between 'reasonable' pharmacological interventions and doping.

Committing to winning and 'realism', 1965–1998

Notwithstanding the medicalisation and scientisation of elite sport described above, French athletes, with a few exceptions, enjoyed relatively little success in major international competitions. In athletics, for example, French throwers used power training and other training techniques similar to foreign athletes but still lagged behind in the medal counts (Singler and Treutlein, 2000: 37). In an attempt to help the nation win more medals, doctors inside the sports world began advocating for more 'realism' and the more liberal use of pharmacology under medical supervision.

The push for 'realism' in France had a strong foreign influence. French newspapers stoked debate and supported medicalising elite sport by publishing statements by West German physicians on the necessity of providing pharmacological support to elite sportspeople. At a conference in Freiburg, Germany, in 1976, Dr Willi Hollmann framed the use of pharmacology in terms of Cold War sports competition:

> There are three possible solutions: either we ban anabolics totally, and in this case, we surrender unconditionally against the Eastern Bloc, or the IOC clears the Olympic program of sports where the use of anabolic steroids is permanent (I know this is true in 18 of the 21 officially registered sports), or else we try to help sportspeople by prescribing anabolic steroids in the form of replacement therapy with the least harm to their health.
>
> (*L'Equipe*, 28 October 1976)

At the same conference, Dr Alois Mader, who had treated East German swimmers before his defection to West Germany, agreed and added that a program of sports pharmacology should be run under medical supervision since 'anabolic steroids are safe when they are administered under strict control' (*Tonus*, 26 July 1976). East Germany, like the Soviet Union before it, had emerged in the Cold War as a sporting superpower engaged in a struggle with West Germany. As we have seen, the Cold War was central to the growth and intensification of international sports, especially the Olympics, during the twentieth century (Rider, 2016). As a result, doctors in West Germany increasingly took a central role in maintaining the health (and enhancing the performances) of their sporting patients who were involved in intense sporting (and political) competition against their brother nation. The West German doctor Helmut Philippi (*L'Equipe*, 28 October 1976) described this situation in a medical conference in Cannes, France:

> We must consider that we are facing a problem of choice in a society where there is always total competition (social, economic, political and sports). It

> is whether we say 'yes' to the sport war: if so, we will have to follow the lead of Eastern Europe. If not, we will continue to be ridiculed in high level competitions.

With a focus on the performance rather than the health of German athletes, Philippi saw medicine as serving the state by providing pharmacological techniques to enhance performance to athletes. This orientation made the West German sports model competitive and generated medals through pharmacological support. The medicalised West German model reached France through newspapers, medical journals, conferences and direct contacts. For instance, a leading French sports physician and elite trainer, who was interviewed during our research on the basis of anonymity, told one of the authors (C. B.) that he discovered 'hormonal rebalancing' during a medical training session in a West German hospital. Given medical debates in the 1960s about biological preparation and their investments in competition, French sports doctors at the highest levels were receptive to the idea of providing pharmacological support to elite sportspeople. In the 1970s, doctors increasingly accepted the goal of making France more competitive internationally and, as part of this, they became more vocal in their support for pharmacology. For example, Dr Bernard Caseris (1976), a physician in the medical team of the Tour de France, took a 'realistic' approach, arguing that making pharmacological support public would keep riders safer:

> Do the riders of the Tour de France abuse drugs? There is no doubt. Riders are most often simple people and don't know what they are doing when using drugs. They influence each other and this increases the doses they use. Since amphetamines are prohibited, they will use any psychostimulant including those that have even more harmful effects. It would be better to revise the rules of the race and allow amphetamines within reasonable doses, five to ten milligrams, for example.

In France, Dr Bruno De Lignières, an endocrinologist who specialised in androgens and female contraception, played a central role in developing the idea of pharmacological support for athletes in the 1970s. In 1975, Pierre Mazeaud, the Youth and Sports Secretary, asked De Lignières to assist Professor Fernand Plas on three different studies. The first study attempted to ascertain the prevalence of doping behaviour among sportspeople. The second study analysed biological variations in prolonged physical efforts (De Lignières et al., 1976).[1] The third study tested the performance of hormonally boosted sportspeople under natural conditions (as opposed to laboratory conditions) in comparison to a placebo group.

Initially, their findings were well received. However, the findings were criticised when they were presented at the 1980 World Games of Medicine in Cannes. Their presentation made an implicit call for pharmacological support by presenting elite sportspeople as sick and in need of (banned) drugs in order to return to a 'normal' hormonal threshold. De Lignières was criticised for having ties to a pharmaceutical laboratory but, despite this criticism, his ideas circulated widely in medical journals, newspapers, on television and in elite sport.

It is important to note that De Lignières was not an outsider or a marginal practitioner within sports medicine; he was joint winner of the 1975 prize of the French Society of Sports Medicine, and he argued throughout his life that doctors should provide pharmacological support in order to maintain an appropriate hormonal balance in elite athletes (De Lignières and Saint-Martin, 1999). De Lignières received support from Dr Jean-Pierre Koralsztein, who was the physician for the successful Béziers rugby team. They argued that because doctors already provided pharmacological support to ameliorate the effects of fatigue on people with physically demanding jobs, such as miners, farmworkers and longshoremen, they should do the same for elite athletes. Together they denounced what they saw as a moralistic fight against doping and advocated hormonal rebalancing to the National Advisory Council on Ethics in 1989. After four years, the Council responded on 18 May 1993; the Council accepted that steroid hormones protected the health of workers in some occupations, but argued that they were not acceptable for sport workers, that is athletes.

In 1979, Professor Gilbert Dreyfus (an endocrinologist at the Hôpital La Pitié in Paris) and Professor Fernand Plas (cardiologist and director of the Sport Institute of the University of Paris) came to a similar view as De Lignières. Although they criticised the use of corticosteroids and androgens as dangerous and unfair, they supported 'hormonal rebalancing' of sportspeople under medical supervision:

> [C]orrecting an existing trouble after a scientific evaluation, restoring the physiological norms, and promoting the return to personal integrity is an authentic medical act … the doctor must give priority to addressing the immediate causes of physiological and psychological disturbances … the administration of a natural anabolic to correct the damage caused by prolonged exertion provides the recipient a better condition to face coming events. When working with circumstances out of the ordinary, such as when an individual, whose job it is, has to ride a bicycle for three weeks with minimal hours of rest, it may be permissible to correct an androgenic deficiency that is scientifically established and, at the same time, he is prepared to face the next step. This raises the issue of equalizing opportunities in competition.
>
> (Gilbert-Dreyfus and Plas, 1979)

Plas justified hormonal rebalancing by defining elite sport as a work setting that presents special occupational hazards. He expressed particular concern about the physiological damage caused from prolonged, intense exertion demanded by elite sport. Professional sportspeople were workers, he reasoned, with different requirements and constraints from amateurs. For example, professional cyclists raced for three continuous weeks during the Tour de France. This presented their doctors with a choice: either denounce the professional activity that creates harmful fatigue, or perform a 'natural' act that addresses the consequences of prolonged fatigue. Guided by his understanding of medical ethics, Plas recommended that doctors prescribe testosterone, a natural substance produced by the body, rather than a synthetic product.

De Lignières, Koralsztein and Plas were not the only doctors who supported hormonal rebalancing from the perspective of occupational risk. Claude-Louis Gallien was a national hammer thrower in the late 1960s, and later became a professor of biology at the University of Paris V, vice-president of the French National Olympic Committee and president of the International University Sports Federation (FISU). Given his background – and particularly his position within the Olympic movement – one might perhaps have expected him to have opposed pharmacological support. However, in the journal of a student sport association in 1987 and in *L'Equipe* in 1988, Gallien argued that although amateur athletes should not use pharmacological products, professionals could engage in hormonal rebalancing, given the occupational harms of elite sport:

> We must be able to administer to [the athlete], if he is ill, all necessary medications, even if they contain 'banned' molecules that may be found in doping control analysis. We should even be able to administer products considered 'doping' in rational and physiological doses to compensate for certain losses generated by intense efforts.
>
> (*L'Equipe*, 25 November 1987: 21)

Dr François Bellocq also advocated hormonal rebalancing to protect the health of athletes. His MD thesis was entitled *Effects of prolonged muscular effort on the adrenal metabolism: application to professional cyclists* (1976) and, as the team physician for the Peugeot cycling team in the 1970s, Bellocq developed a medical facility for riders that was, at the time, new to professional cycling. His centre also treated international athletes in many sports. Bellocq believed that the goal of sports medicine should be to lead elite sportspeople to the highest attainable standard of health (i.e. maximal capacity for performance). Bellocq rejected the link between elite sport and good health. He saw the intensity of training in elite sport as creating hormonal imbalances in the human body. Disciplines such as cycling and athletics created strong physiological imbalances that need to be offset by 'physiological' doses of cortisone and testosterone. If these readjustments were made scientifically, in small doses and only occasionally, then it would not, he argued, constitute doping since he equated doping with large doses (Bellocq, 1976).

In his book *Le Dopage* (1990), the Belgian sports doctor Dr André Noret, the medical officer for the Union Cycliste Internationale (UCI) World Championships, criticised the moral censure that cyclists received for using drugs while people throughout society use a wide range of drugs, for example, nicotine, alcohol, tranquilisers, ephedrine. He argued that his patients, that is elite cyclists, had extremely low hormone levels that constituted a medical condition of hormonal deficiency. It was, therefore, necessary to administer hormones since it is the physician's role to 'treat according to the rules of the art of healing and the Code of Medical Ethics' (Noret, 1990: 193). For example, sports doctors regularly prescribed iron, magnesium or potassium when the patient had a deficit of these substances. So, he asked, why not prescribe hormones too? By making pharmacology part of a healthy training regime, Noret placed the sports doctor at the heart of 'the triangle of success' alongside the athlete and coach.

We should note, however, that the 'triangle of success' was reserved for male athletes. Noret argued that 'androgen therapy should be forbidden to sportswomen' (Noret, 1990). Given his 'realist', less moral perspective, Noret's opposition to hormonal rebalancing for sportswomen may seem inconsistent with his support for the hormonal rebalancing of sportsmen. What we see here is a gendered morality imposed upon the bodies of sportswomen. Dr Stanislas Burstin (federal doctor of the cycling and football federations) called female contraception 'cheating nature' (Burstin, 1965). Similarly, Dr Catherine Defoligny (director of the Medical Office of the Youth and Sport Ministry and a former international fencer) wondered if the contraceptive pill that could 'get rid of troublesome menstrual events on the occasion of a competition' respected the ethics of sport (Defoligny, 1980: 30). We see here once again that admixture of medical/scientific knowledge on the one hand and value-laden, extra-scientific social-moral values on the other, an ever-present and problematic characteristic of modern sports medicine from its early beginnings. The central concern of these, mostly male, doctors was the visible femininity of sportswomen. In the 1970s and 1980s, close-up colour television pictures allowed viewers to see the highly developed musculature of champion sportswomen. Anxiety about the effects of pharmacology on sportswomen's bodies reached its apogee when East German swimmers showed signs of virilisation (facial hair, reduced fat, low voice). The invocation of female athletes' bodies masculinised by pharmacology was a gendered ideology which presented pharmacology – but only as applied to female athletes – as an affront to nature while deflecting attention away from the artificiality of intensive training. The imposition of a gendered morality upon sportswomen illustrates how pharmacology and bodily stereotyping were wedded together in the policing of athletes' bodies (Bohuon, 2015: 969).

In this chapter we have seen that the growing involvement of physicians in sport created serious conflicts within the role of the sports physician. Sports physicians were, to varying degrees, caught between the demands of their codes of medical ethics, the goal of sporting success at the elite level and the unsafe demands of intensive sports training and competition. The ambiguities within sports medicine threw up important questions which they could hardly avoid. What was their proper role as doctors? Should they ban unsafe products even though the continued illicit use of these products without medical supervision would make elite sport even more unhealthy? Or should they supervise these practices to mitigate risks to the health of sportspeople? As we have seen, many doctors argued that athletes should be permitted to use, under medical supervision, substances normally regarded as doping. From the 1960s to the late 1990s, the use of pharmacology in elite sport expanded enormously under the banner of 'hormonal rebalancing', and as a result of the Festina affair in the 1998 Tour de France, the reality of the widespread use of pharmacological products in professional cycling – and the role of team doctors in this process – became headline news around the world. We examine this issue in the case study in the next chapter.

Note

1 We have been unable to find the results of these studies but we learned from interviewing ten participants in the research that 70 per cent of the participants reported having used performance-enhancing drugs.

References

Ballester, P. (2015), Rugby à charge. L'enquête choc, Paris, De la Martinière.

Bellocq, F. (1976), *Effets des efforts musculaires prolongés sur le métabolisme surréna: application aux coureurs cyclistes professionnels,* MD Thesis, University of Bordeaux.

Bellocq, F. and Bressan, S. (1991), *Sport et dopage: La grande hypocrisie,* Paris, Du Félin.

Bohuon, A. (2015), Gender Verifications in Sport: From an East/West Antagonism to a North/South Antagonism, *International Journal of the History of Sport*, 32 (7), 965–979.

Boissier, J-R. (1964), Présentation. Premier colloque européen sur le doping et la préparation biologique du sportif de compétition, January 26–27 1963, Uriage les Bains, Medecine, *Education et Sport*, 1, 18–21.

Brissonneau, C. (2003), *Entrepreneurs de morale et carrières de deviants dans le dopage sportif: prises de position et témoignages vécus dans la médecine du sport et dans deux disciplines sportives, l'athlétisme et le cyclisme sur la route (1960–2003)*, Ph Dissertation, Paris X Nanterre University.

Burger, R. (1967), Quo vadis…sport cycliste? *Le Miroir du cyclisme,* 92, 6–7.

Burstin S. (1965), *Contribution à l'étude du dopage professionnel*, Paris, Lille.

Caseris, B. (1976), Revue Tonus, 26 juillet.

Coakley, J. (2009), *Sports in Society: Issues and Controversies*, 10th ed., Boston, McGraw Hill.

Crespin, M. (1968), Lettre du Colonel Marceau Crespin, *Médecine du Sport,* 4, 4–25.

Delezenne, L. (1963), Considérations actuelles sur le doping, *Médecine, éducation physique et sport,* 4, 32–38.

Defoligny, C. (1980), Le Sport Féminin et ses aspects médicaux, Revue EP&S, 163, 28–31.

Defoligny, C. (1981), Où en est la médecine du sport en France, *Médecine du sport*, 55 (5), 4–5.

De Lignières, B., et al. (1976), Variations plasmatiques des androgènes et du cortisol au cours des efforts physiques prolongés. *Médecine du sport*, 50(3), 7–16.

De Lignières, B. and Saint-Martin, E. (1999), *Vive le dopage?: Enquête sur un alibi,* Paris, Flammarion.

Dreyfus, G. and Plas, F. (1979), Sur l'emploi des substances hormonales dans la pratique sportive, *Bulletin de l'Académie nationale de médecine*, 163, 73–78.

Duchesnay, G. (1959), Orientations de la préthérapeutique des états de la fatigue, *Médecine, éducation physique et sport,* 6, 293–297.

Guillet, R. (1964), *Le doping de l'homme et du cheval,* Paris, Masson.

La Cava, G. (1954), Le 'doping'. *Médecine, éducation physique et sport,* 1, 24–27.

Le Breton, D. (2010), *Expériences de la douleur*, Paris, Métailié.

Lemarchands, H. (1964), Présentation. Premier colloque européen sur le doping et la préparation biologique du sportif de compétition, 26–27 January 1963, *Uriage les Bains*, 1, 21–24.

Miserez, P. (1976), Dopage. Les révélations d'un médecin du Tour, *Sports Magazine*, 2, 7 July–27 August.

Noret, A. (1990), *Le dopage,* Paris, Vigot.

Palliere, J. (1964), Présentation. *Premier colloque européen sur le doping et la préparation biologique du sportif de compétition,* 26–27 January 1963, *Uriage les Bains*, 1, 39–42.

Rapport de la Commission des athlètes (1964), Premier colloque européen sur le doping et la préparation biologique du sportif de compétition, 26–27 January 1963, Uriage les Bains, *Médecine, Education et Sport*, 1, 50–52.
Rider, T. C. (2016), *Cold War Games: Propaganda, the Olympics, and U.S. Foreign Policy*, Urbana-Champagne, University of Illinois Press.
Rouanet, S. (2014), *Dans la peau d'un athlète*, Paris, Armand Collin.
Singler, A. and Treutlein, G. (2000), *Doping im Spitzensport: Sportwissenschaftliche Analysen zur nationalen und internationalen Leistungentwicklung*, Aachen, Meyer & Meyer.

10 Drug use in elite sport

A case study of professional cycling and the 1998 Tour de France

We have argued in previous chapters that a number of key themes can be identified in the development of modern sports medicine from its early origins. These include: (i) an early focus on sport rather than on public health issues; (ii) this early focus on sport became increasingly a focus on elite, competitive sport; (iii) sports physicians became increasingly involved in, and central to, the networks of relationships surrounding elite athletes; (iv) within these networks, doctors became increasingly involved in the search for enhanced performances; and (v) that for a significant number of sports physicians, the search for enhanced performance came to include an acceptance of the use of performance-enhancing drugs. The object of this chapter is to show, via a case study of the development of professional cycling in the second half of the twentieth century, and in particular the scandal involving organised, systematic and widespread doping in the 1998 Tour de France, how these processes developed within one particular professional sport. Although each sport has its own special features, the general pattern of development in cycling – and particularly the increasing involvement of team doctors/sports physicians in the search for enhanced performance – is typical of the development of modern sport in general.

After the scandal in the 1998 Tour de France – the so-called Festina affair, named after the team at the heart of the scandal – many key actors within professional cycling broke their silence to explain what had become the normality of doping in cycling; in effect, the Festina scandal opened up a space for discussion in which many of those engaged in cycling felt able to speak out publicly. One consequence for researchers was that it became possible to speak with cycling 'insiders' about a topic that had, for a long time, been taboo. This presented one of the authors (C.B.) with the opportunity to interview elite cyclists and doctors in France about drug use in professional cycling and this chapter includes data from these interviews.

Before we examine the social processes at the heart of the Festina affair, it may be useful to note briefly some of the major doping scandals in cycling in France in the twentieth century.

DOI: 10.4324/9781003563921-14

Doping scandals before the Festina affair

Drug use in professional cycling has a long history. What Richard Williams, writing in *The Guardian* (1 August 1998), described as cycling's 'intimate association with doping' can be traced back a long way. In the late nineteenth century, riders in the six-day races used a mixture of heroin and cocaine to increase endurance. In 1924 the Pelissier brothers, in a famous interview with the investigative journalist Albert Londres, described the physical demands which the Tour de France made on the riders and the drugs which they used. The interview took place on the eve of a Tour stage on 27 June 1924:

> Do you want to see what we run on? Look'. From his bag [Henri] took out a phial: 'That's cocaine for our eyes, that's chloroform for the gums'. 'That', said Ville, also emptying his *musette*, is a cream to warm up my knees'. 'And the pills, do you want to see the pills? Look, here are the pills'. They each took out three boxes. 'In short', said Francis, we run on "dynamite" '.
>
> (cited in Mignon, 2003: 230)

More recently, the first five men in the 1966 World Road Race championship all refused to take a drugs test; the five included Jaques Anquetil, five times winner of the Tour de France, who later admitted to taking stimulants and said: 'Everyone in cycling dopes himself and those who claim they do not are liars' (*The Times*, 21 July 1988).

In the 1976 'Courrier de Dax', a local race at the end of the 1976 season, two riders picked for drug control at random, Rachel Dard and Bernard Bourreau, tried to elude the doping tests. Being unable to evade the test, they each had to provide a urine sample. One of the cyclists, Dard, together with a cycling colleague, followed the doctor who had collected the sample onto the train to Paris. After a discussion on the train, these cyclists persuaded the doctor to throw the sample down the drain; the incident became common knowledge and made headline news. The French cycling federation sanctioned all the participants in this affair (Vincent, 1976).

Several important cases hit the cycling world during the 1980s. One of the most important was that of the 'Six Days of Bercy', an indoor race in Paris held in a small velodrome in November 1986. The police unit responsible for fighting drug dealing raided this event and arrested dealers of amphetamines (*Le Monde*, 19 November 1986, Descentes et poursuites. available at: https://www.lemonde.fr/archives/article/1986/11/19/descente-et-poursuites_2926959_1819218.html). The following year, in October 1987, at Laon, 62 people (20 cyclists, 19 doctors, 23 chemists) belonging to a doping network of drug providers/users were prosecuted (*Le Monde*, Des sportifs et leurs médecins en correctionnelle. 13 October 1987).

It is important to make the point that the fact that drug use in professional cycling – and indeed in many other sports – has a long history going back to before the development of modern sports medicine means that one cannot say in any simple sense that the use of drugs in sport was 'caused' by the development of sports medicine. However, as we will see, the case study of cycling shows very clearly that the increasing involvement of sports physicians as team doctors in professional cycling was associated with a marked change in the *pattern* of drug use in cycling.

The 1998 Tour de France: l'Affaire Festina

As we noted earlier, the team at the heart of the Tour de France scandal was Festina, whose masseur, Willy Voet, was arrested *en route* to the start of the Tour when French police found 250 batches of anabolic steroids and 400 ampoules of erythropoietin (EPO) in his car. Although the Tour organisers originally tried to play down the significance of Voet's arrest, suggesting that he may have been working on his own without the knowledge of the team, it quickly emerged that there was, within the Festina team, an organised and systematic programme of drug use by team members. Under police questioning, the team director admitted to French police that 'a concerted system for supplying cyclists with drugs was organised between management, doctors, the masseur and the riders', and following this admission, the whole team was expelled from the race (*Sunday Times*, 19 July 1998).

More revelations about drug taking came out on an almost daily basis and it became increasingly clear that the highly organised system of drug use revealed in the Festina team was also characteristic of most other professional teams. The French police also took an increasingly prominent role in the Tour, searching the hotels and vehicles of several teams and taking riders to hospital to require them to give blood, hair and urine samples for drug testing. Riders protested against the police actions by sitting down in the road and refusing to race. Most riders were eventually persuaded to continue the race but three teams withdrew from the race. By the end of the Tour, police had found banned drugs in the hotels or vehicles used by four teams, Festina, TVM, ONCE and Casino. Eventually fewer than half the riders finished the race, largely because several teams were either suspended from the race or withdrew in connection with the allegations concerning drug use (Waddington, 2000: 156–159).

One of the difficulties in studying patterns of drug use in sport concerns the difficulty of getting reliable information. It is for this reason that events such as the 1998 Tour de France are so important for researchers, for they provide a wealth of information about drug use which those involved in the use of drugs normally try to keep secret. In this regard, the 1998 Tour marked a landmark in the study of drug use in sport not just because of the huge quantity but, perhaps even more importantly, because of the reliable quality of the data which was made publicly available by the media and, later, by the court cases arising from the arrests of several key actors in the Tour drama. It may therefore be useful to reflect on some of the central issues to come out of the 1998 Tour scandal.

Perhaps the key point to be made is that the revelations from the 1998 Tour bring out in a particularly clear way the figuration of relationships among those involved in what has been called the 'doping network' (Waddington, 2000: 159). In this regard, it should be noted that, following the police investigation, not only were several of the world's leading cyclists charged by French police with offences under France's anti-doping laws but – perhaps more significantly – other key actors in the doping network, including three team doctors, three masseurs and two team directors, were also identified and charged under the anti-doping laws. When placed alongside other detailed and reliable case studies, such as those provided by the Dubin Commission of Canada's 1988 Olympic weightlifting and sprint teams (Dubin, 1990: 139–176; 234–259), it is clear that, at the elite level, it is simply unrealistic to see the individual drug-using athlete as working alone, without the assistance and support of others with specialised knowledge and expertise.

It is therefore important not to focus exclusively on the individual athlete, for it is important to recognise that it is not only the athletes who may perceive their best interests to be served by the use of performance-enhancing drugs, for doctors, team managers, coaches, officials and others may also, for whatever reasons – career advancement, national prestige or financial gain, for example – perceive their best interests to be served by encouraging or concealing, or at least 'turning a blind eye' to, the illicit use of drugs. This is, it might be suggested, one of the primary reasons why the use of performance-enhancing drugs has proved so difficult to control. Although we are not concerned here to examine the (in)effectiveness of anti-doping policy (that has been done elsewhere; see, for example, Waddington and Smith, 2009; Waddington, 2019; Waddington and Møller, 2019; Moston and Engelberg, 2017), it is clear that if we hope to develop a more effective anti-drugs policy, then that policy will have to be based on considerably more than a narrowly technological approach, concerned simply with developing more sophisticated testing techniques, that we need to move away from the almost exclusive focus on the individual drug-using athlete and that we need to take into account the complexities of the social networks in which athletes are involved and in which sports physicians are, all too frequently, major actors. In the following section we analyse these changing patterns of relationships – that is, the structure of the 'doping networks' – and the central role of team doctors, in modern cycling.

Drug use in French cycling in the modern era

Brissonneau (2000, 2015) has identified what may be described as two modes of production of the cycling performance, the first of which characterised professional cycling in France until the 1980s, while the second developed from the mid-1980s. Each mode of production is characterised by a particular pattern of relationships between those involved in producing the cycling performance and, importantly, each mode of production is associated with a distinctive pattern of drug use.

Empiricism and dabbling in drugs (1960–1980s)

Until the mid-1980s, the mode of production of the cycling performance may be described as artisanal. Sponsorship deals were relatively small and teams were small in size, composed of no more than 20 people, including the cyclists. Staff consisted mostly of family members and former riders, all of whom shared a past history in cycling. There was a simple division of labour with relatively little specialisation. Labour was divided equally among staff members and tasks were shared. At the head of the team, the team director (*directeur sportif*), was a former cyclist who had many functions including those of manager and trainer. He also liaised with sponsors, recruited team members and hired mechanics and soigneurs (also former cyclists) who helped with everyday jobs such as washing clothes and cleaning bikes. The *directeur sportif* also created the race schedule. The team was paid to represent the sponsor as much as possible and, for this reason, cyclists rode a lot of races, perhaps as many as two or three races each week in the spring and summer. The Tour de France was the central objective but only became the focal point a few weeks prior to the race.

Training was empirically based and the same all year round. In marked contrast to modern training systems, it also reflected an emphasis on quantity rather than quality, with riders typically riding long distances in training day after day; there was no question of honing one's fitness according to a carefully worked-out plan. 'Training meant riding like crazy. It meant never riding short distances, never just riding kilometres but piling them up' (Eric, 1970s rider).

Few cyclists worked with a doctor or specialised trainer and the evaluation of their training programme was empirical; training was not monitored on the basis of the systematic collection of biological data, but was based on feeling, sensations, and the whims of the moment. Subject to deep fatigue due to physical effort and travel, the use of drugs was commonplace. Amphetamines were used to combat fatigue for one or two hours, during the race, and sometimes during hard training.

Amphetamines were also used to fight fatigue associated with travel between criteriums. These races, commonly held in July after the Tour de France, are the times when cyclists could earn a lot of money, often representing 50% of their annual salary.

> Our team might take stimulants that are on the banned list. But it was not for the race. The result was not of paramount importance. It was for the long and tiring hours in the car and the driving that went along with it. Because we had to take long trips during this period of racing criteriums. [...] In those circumstances it was not the cyclists who doped, but the driver of the car.
>
> (Bastide, 1970: 173)

Steroids (cortisone, anabolic steroids) relieved the deep fatigue of long periods of training, racing and travelling and allowed heavier training loads, even though the use of drugs was unsystematic. As one informant explained about the effect of corticosteroids:

> It's the evening when you come back, you ride 150 km in training, with normal muscle aches. You can train again the morning of the next day! That's the difference. Usually, after two months in season, when you come back from training, when you come back from races, you can't ride hard again the next day. You can't do intensive work. But with those things!
>
> (Eric, 1970s rider)

Already the use of drugs was considered to be a medical technique, something which helped to optimise performance. It was not considered as a way to cheat, that is to say, to illegally gain an unfair advantage over other cyclists (Brissonneau, 2007: 136). In this regard, it is important to emphasise that cyclists are not immoral; they have ethical standards and conventions relating to professional cycling – for example, riders do not take what is considered an unfair advantage if the race leader has to stop for a 'natural break' – but in their world, drugs were not considered as cheating but as a medically based way to optimise work performance. 'A cheater is one who clings to the door of a car or someone who takes a shortcut, but doping?' (Bastide, 1970: 185).

Drugs were often self-administered and riders obtained their drugs from a variety of sources; drugs might be obtained from sharing with other riders, from drug dealers, from chemists and sometimes from local doctors who, fascinated by elite sport, also participated in the doping process.

Alain (1970s rider):	I went to the corner pharmacy with the prescription that the doctor had given me, and it's the nurse who gave me the injections as prescribed by the doctor. And I had the doctor's prescription. I said, 'You give it to me, you inject it'.
Interviewer:	Why did he give it to you? He sold it to you?
Alain:	Not really. They are not trying to take advantage of you. They do it to help

Although the use of drugs was widespread, their use was unsystematic and was not integrated into a scientifically constructed training programme. Consistent with the empiricist approach to training, this period was characterised by what might be called dabbling in drugs, rather than the scientific use of drugs as part of a systematic training programme.

This mode of production of the cycling performance – small scale, artisanal and based on small budgets and family support – increasingly gave way from the beginning of the 1980s to a better financed and more highly rationalised system based on an increasingly scientific approach to training.

A new mode of performance production

From the mid-1980s, cycling entered a new era with an economic boom in the cycling market characterised by spectacularisation and by a reorganisation of cycle racing by the sport's governing bodies, together with increased TV coverage of the Tour (see Brewer, 2002; Lagrue, 2004). These changes in the cycling market generated higher levels of sponsorship from major international companies and a change in the management of teams, with a movement away from the artisanal, family style of management towards a modern enterprise style of management. These changes were also associated with changes in performance standards and in the mode of production of the sporting performance, including the size and structure of the teams, the specialisation of labour and organisation of training and competition, and the pattern and organisation of drug usage.

In the 1970s, fewer spectators had been watching the Tour de France, whether at the roadside or on TV. Two Tour directors, Jacques Goddet and Felix Levitan, sought to revive interest in the spectacle of cycling by developing the internationalisation of the competitors (most riders at that time were from Western Europe). This increase in the geographical diversity of the competitors was designed to rekindle the enthusiasm of spectators and attract them back to watching the Tour. It was for this reason that they turned to the American continent (Louy, 2007), which also represented a huge potential market for the declining French cycling industry. The inclusion of Americans, most notably the future Tour de France winner, Greg Lemond, opened a new chain of recruitment for European teams.

Goddet and Levitan also tried to attract the best Olympic amateur riders from Eastern Europe. These high-performance riders were less expensive and were recruited by European teams after the fall of the Berlin Wall in 1989. They also came with a new scientific vision of training and a knowledge of doping gleaned from the state-sponsored doping programmes in some Eastern European countries.

Also in the 1980s, the privatisation of the French TV channels had an impact. Private TV channels needed to fill many hours of programming and turned to sports shows which were less costly to produce. They broadcast hundreds of hours of cycling, with a focus on the Tour de France. This attracted new national and international sponsors who saw the possibility of many hours of relatively low cost exposure to large numbers of TV spectators. Those new sponsors injected a great deal of money into cycling but in return, they sought to optimise their investment. This involved targeting the most important races with a central focus on the prestigious Tour de France.

These changes were associated with a transition in the management model within teams. Cycling teams that up to that point had been organised on limited budgets and according to a family management model moved increasingly towards an enterprise model of management with considerably enlarged budgets. One of the key changes was at the level of staffing. The team director no longer did everything, but became the team manager with responsibility for finding sponsors, recruiting and supervising staff members. Previously, team directors had had a more or less close link with cycling and undertook a variety of tasks associated with team management. Now each staff member was required to have a more specialised competence in a specific role as part of the rationalisation process within the team. Imposed by those new managerial actors, a more formalised division of labour developed within professional teams. One of the consequences was that, within teams, riders became more specialised (climbers, sprinters, lead-out riders); these specialists were required to perform not only during a specific part of the race (e.g. in the mountains) but also to assist their team leader. In return, teammates were paid well for a job that might otherwise have seemed unglamourous.

When we asked support riders if they had no ambition of their own, they appeared content with the situation of being a support rider even though this meant it was beyond their reach to achieve much success on a personal level. As one rider explained:

> There are ambitions but a professional rider knows he doesn't have the opportunity to win the Tour de France or a beautiful Classic. So ... it's the personal satisfaction of having worked for a leader, to have done the maximum possible. It is self-sacrifice.
>
> (Mickaël, rider in the 1980s)

Because of these changes, new people, outsiders to the traditional cycling family, arrived. In order to optimise training methods and the team's potential, team managers recruited doctors and other scientists such as specialists in exercise physiology. They were employed by team directors in order to improve the riders' health and to focus on certain races, with the most important being the Tour de France. In the 1970s doctors with an interest in cycling might 'help' individual cyclists by prescribing drugs for them, but doctors were not generally integrated into the team structure. By the 1990s, the major professional teams all had team doctors and other scientists who became increasingly important in drawing up training programmes and in monitoring cyclists' health and performance. Cyclists too came to understand the importance of the input from sports physicians, attending sports medicine departments where they did maximum cardiac effort tests to determine their different work phases and had blood tests to evaluate their fatigue level. The body came to be considered like a motor engine composed of fluid levels. Pharmaceutical products were considered as regulators when levels became too low. Team doctors planned training loads several months in advance in order for the cyclists to peak at particular times and for particular races. With the impact of this more intensive scientific training, the cyclists we interviewed described a significant increase in pain, injuries and fatigue. That is why words such as 'health', 'take care of' or 'recovery' became ubiquitous among cyclists. In 'taking care' of the cyclists' health – a euphemism for drug use – the relationship between riders and sports physicians became increasingly important.

Another consequence of critical importance was the mediation of doctors between riders and biological knowledge. Whereas under the artisanal style of management, the riders themselves had sourced and largely self-administered the drugs which they used, with the development of larger and better resourced teams with their own medical and scientific support teams, the purchase of the drugs was centrally organised while the drugs were administered and the riders monitored by team physicians. For example, following the revelations of widespread doping at the 1998 Tour de France, Bruno Roussel, the Festina team director, told police that since 1993, when he had taken over as team director, the team had maintained a 'war chest' of 400,000 francs (about £40,000) (or about 1 per cent of the team's annual budget of £4 million), the money being siphoned off from the cash paid out by the team to riders to reward good performances (Waddington, 2000: 156–157). The objective, he said, 'was to improve performances under strict medical control in order to avoid the unauthorised personal supply to cyclists causing grave attacks on their health which could have been the case in the past' (*Sunday Telegraph*, 19 July 1998). Thus whereas riders had previously self-administered drugs based on little more than the shared lay knowledge of other riders, team physicians were now able to prescribe precise doses, based on systematic biological data obtained from each rider, and therefore geared to the individual requirements of each rider. It might be noted that Roussel's argument – that control of the doping process by team physicians reduced the risk of more dangerous use of drugs by riders in an uncontrolled fashion – was one which, as we saw in previous chapters, had frequently been used by sports physicians for very many years. As Roussel implied, whereas riders had previously dabbled in drugs such as amphetamines and steroids, their training and racing was now increasingly based on the systematic use of drugs which was fully integrated into a scientific training programme under the control of team physicians. One can see here very clearly what Fincoeur (2016: 206, cited in Paoli, 2019: 85) has described as the 'medicalisation of doping', that is the increasing sophistication of the doping process and its integration within a comprehensive scientific training programme.

A comparison between the training regime of professional riders under the artisanal system and after the systematic incorporation of doctors and other scientists in training and racing programmes from the 1980s is very instructive. Louison Bobet was a three-time winner of the Tour de France and the training schedule he used in 1957 shows the largely quantitative nature of training prior to the involvement of sports physicians and other scientists in cycling from the 1980s (see Table 10.1, from Marchand, 1963: 65). It is a six-week training schedule in which the days and weeks are largely undifferentiated except to keep track of the distance ridden on any given day during training. It also tracks the distance ridden each week and the total distance ridden over the six-week period. While the schedule appears superficially rational, it is in fact simply a training diary which tracks the distance he had ridden. In effect, Bobet simply rode his bike, with the distances increasing week by week, and logged the kilometres.

In marked contrast is the training schedule provided to us by one of our interviewees, Nicolas, who had been a professional rider in the 1990s. In the first two decades of the twentieth century training programmes for professional cyclists were to become considerably more sophisticated than Nicolas's programme from the 1990s, with a clear differentiation between training for speed, power and/or endurance (see, e.g., the training programme of Davide Rebellin, in Brissoneau and Montez de Oca, 2018: 91). Nevertheless, Nicolas's training programme, set out in Table 10.2, is very different from that of Bobet because, unlike Bobet's programme, it is not a simple training programme but an integrated *training and doping programme* and, as such, it provides a clear indication of the passage from empirical training, based on sensations, to a more scientific approach in which everything (training and pharmacology) is calibrated.

In this chart, we see how the sports physician and other biological scientists and the trainer combine, with their roles becoming complementary (training time and gear ratios, monitoring heart rate, providing and monitoring effects of drugs). Those scientists managed all physical facets of training and competing.

Table 10.1 Louison Bobet's six-week training schedule (kilometres), 1957

	Monday	*Tuesday*	*Wednesday*	*Thursday*	*Friday*	*Saturday*	*Sunday*	*Total*
Week 1	20	30	30	50	30	50	50	260
Week 2	20	60	30	70	50	80	50	360
Week 3	20	70	50	80	80	30	80	410
Week 4	20	80	50	100	50	20	100	420
Week 5	20	80	50	140	30	20	120	460
Week 6	20	80	50	140	30	0	0	320
Total kilometres								2230

Table 10.2 Nicolas's scientific training-doping programme

Day	*Training time*	*Heart rate*	*Gear ratio*	*Dosage*	*Time of injection*
M	4 h	145–155	53 x 16	1 GH IM	19 h
T	4 h	130–145	53 x 18	1 GH IM	19 h
W	Rest	1 lipostadil IM			
T	4 h	130–145	53 x 18	1 GH IM	19 h
F	4 h	155–165	53 x 16	1/2 GH SC	17 h

HG = Growth hormone IM = Intra Muscular SC = Subcutaneous Injection

And associated with this, control of coaching within elite cycling teams shifted away from traditional coaches and team directors and towards physicians and other sports scientists.

This shift in power away from traditional coaches and towards sports physicians and sports scientists was nicely described by Antoine Vayer, a former coach to the Festina team. Vayer explained that it was difficult to challenge the growing influence of team doctors: 'Progressively, I understood why they told me, in 1997, "It is not the best coach in the world on the best team in the world that we have now, but the best doctor"'. Vayer said that, even as coach, he was excluded from the riders' meetings when they discussed 'care', but he 'still knew what was going on'. And he described how his more traditional training programme for the riders was increasingly replaced by a medically controlled training programme in which drug use was a central element:

> From September 1997, I started looking more closely at the 'dosages' … When a guy says to you after two years of quality training, 'Now you piss me off with your sets, it needs to develop. So now I have a packed cell volume of 53 when I measured it this morning on my machine; I ride 200km, at my maximum, behind the moped with three fruit pastries and that's it! I recovered with a [IV] drip. My blood drops to 48 with a Clenbuterol [anabolic steroid] cure coupled with growth hormones and it gives me all of the strength I lack' … I have measured the magnitude then and since. And I calculated it all. Incredible. Instead of training at '350 watts' as before when they had some problems with my training, they trained at '400 watts' and rode at the front of the group, and were recovering better and better while being psychologically euphoric.
>
> (Martel and Watbled, 2005)

The information which emerged as a result of the action by the French police during the 1998 Tour de France indicated very clearly that the system at Festina was not unique, but was also found in other professional teams. For example, while the team doctor at Festina, Erik Rijkaert, was arrested and charged under the 1989 Anti-Drug Act, so too were Andrei Mikhailov, who was the doctor of the TVM team, and Nicholas Torralbos, team doctor of the ONCE team.

Professional cycling in the United States

Doctors in cycling teams based outside of Europe were also closely involved in the training and 'preparation' of riders and it is clear that the prosecutions associated with the 1998 Tour de France did not break the increasingly close relationship between cyclists and doctors in the search for enhanced performance. In his autobiography, Tyler Hamilton, who rode with Lance Armstrong at the US Postal Team, but who also took drugs when riding with other teams, recalled that 'it had felt like an honour to be asked to dope by the team doctor', because it meant that he was in line to be selected to ride the Tour de France (Hamilton and Coyle, 2012: 253). And asked by his co-author how he avoided testing positive for so many years, Hamilton replied: 'The tests are easy to beat. We're way, way ahead of the tests. They've got their doctors and we've got ours, and ours are better. Better paid, for sure' (ibid: 10). Elsewhere he said that 'If you were careful and paid attention, you could dope and be 99 per cent certain that you would not get caught … all you had to do was to follow the team doctor's instructions' (ibid: 136).

The centrality of doctors – and of drugs – in the training of elite cyclists is nicely brought home by Hamilton in his description of the training and preparation of riders in the CSC-Tiscali team, which he joined after leaving Armstrong's US Postal team. Hamilton was introduced by his new *directeur sportif*, Bjarni Riis, to a Spanish doctor, Eufemiano Fuentes. Significantly, Hamilton described Fuentes as 'the man who would define the next few years of my life'; we can best understand what Hamilton meant by this if we bear in mind that, as we saw in Chapter 6, Fuentes was at the time running an extensive 'blood doping' network for elite athletes, including many cyclists.

Writing of his time with Lance Armstrong's team, Hamilton recalled that in early season races Armstrong would talk to riders from other teams to get as much information as possible about the fitness and progress of his likely Tour de France rivals. So he would ask: 'What was going on, what was new? How did Ulrich look? How was Pantani climbing?' And, most significantly, 'What doctors were they working with?' (ibid: 141). And when the investigation by the US Anti-Doping Agency finally revealed the extent of organised drug use on Armstrong's team – not just EPO but also blood transfusions, testosterone, corticosteroids and masking agents – it also revealed, once more, the central role of doctors in the doping process, with the investigation generating 'more than enough evidence to proceed with charges' against three of Armstrong's former team doctors, Pedro Celaya, Luis Garcia del Moral and, most significantly, Professor Michel Ferrari, in the doping process (USADA, 2012: 4).

Fatigue and drug use revisited

In the previous chapter we examined the importance of fatigue as a key limitation on performance and the relationship between fatigue and the search for drugs which can help to overcome the effects of fatigue. This case study of cycling provides an appropriate point to revisit the relationship between fatigue – and the associated pain and suffering – and the provision (by team doctors) and the use (by professional cyclists) of drugs. In this context, Mignon (2003: 207) has written that 'there are a lot of good reasons … to find doping in the Tour de France because it is such a hard race that it pushes the sport of cycling … to extremes'.

Earlier in this chapter, we quoted from the famous interview between the journalist Albert Londres and the Pelissier brothers during the 1924 Tour de France, in which they described the drugs they used. But the brothers also emphasised that their drug use was a response to the huge physical demands of the Tour:

> 'You have no idea what the Tour de France is' said Henri. 'It's a Calvary. Worse: the road to the Cross has only14 stations: ours has 15. We suffer from start to finish'…
>
> Henri continued: 'You haven't seen us in the bath after the finish. Buy a ticket for the show. When we've got the mud off, we're white as a funeral shroud, drained empty by diarrhoea; we pass out in the water. At night, in the bedroom, we can't sleep, we twitch and dance and jig about like St Vitus …
>
> 'There's less flesh on our bodies than you'd see on a skeleton', said Francis.
>
> 'And our toe nails', said Henri, 'I've lost six out of ten, they get worn away bit by bit every stage' [from pressure from the toeclips].
>
> 'They grow back next year', said his brother …
>
> 'So, that's it. And you've seen nothing yet; you wait until the Pyrenees, that's "hard labour" '.
>
> (Londres, 1999 [1924]: 16)

It is interesting to note that Londres had first come to prominence as an investigative journalist when he revealed the extremely harsh conditions in the penal colonies in French Guyana and, in his 1924 series of 11 articles on the Tour de France, he compared the physical demands made on the cyclists to the demands made on the criminals condemned to hard labour in those colonies; significantly, his 11 articles were published under the heading 'The Tour of Suffering'.

Suffering – that is fatigue and sheer physical exhaustion – remains a major problem with which professional cyclists (and their team doctors) have to deal. Writing in *The Guardian* (1 August 1998) shortly after the 1998 Tour de France, Richard Williams, noted that:

> As Chris Boardman, the British cyclist … once said: 'It's painful, it's dangerous, and it goes on a long time'. And in a sense, bicycle racers use drugs not to go faster but merely to take away the pain.

There is however an important difference between the causes of the exhaustion and suffering of the Pelissier brothers and the exhaustion of modern Tour riders. As the Pelissier brothers made clear, their fatigue and the associated physical and psychological suffering, as well as their use of drugs to combat the fatigue, was a consequence of the huge distances they were required to ride. Of the 15 stages in the 1924 Tour de France – or, as they put it, of the 15 'stations to Calvary' – only 2 were less than 300 kilometres in length, while there were 6 stages of over 400 kilometres, with the longest stage being 482 kilometres. While the modern Tour de France has more stages – in 2023 there were 21 stages – these are very much shorter than in the Pelissier's Tour of 1924. In 2023, there were only 2 stages longer than 200 kilometres, with the longest stage being 208 kilometres. In 1924 the Tour covered a total of 5,524 kilometres, at an average distance of 368 kilometres per stage; in 2023, the Tour covered 3,381 kilometres at an average of 161 kilometres per stage.

Although riders in the modern Tour de France cover much less distance than the riders in the 1920s, that does not mean that the Tour is now less physically demanding or painful for the riders; indeed it is clear that the Tour remains a huge physical (and psychological) challenge for riders. However, the source of the riders' exhaustion is now rather different from the source of the exhaustion of the Pelissier brothers. The critical point here is that while riders of earlier generations rode very long distances in both training and racing – Louison Bobet's training diary, it will be recalled, indicated that his training simply consisted of riding as much and as far as he could – modern elite cyclists spend less time simply riding long distances but, under the watchful eyes of their sports physicians, they follow a carefully worked-out scientific programme which involves training at a much higher level of intensity which is designed specifically to subject their bodies to stresses in order to build up strength, which, in turn, enables them to race at much higher levels of intensity.

And it is clear that, whatever the sources of the riders' pain, the Tour remains an exhausting experience. An 'insider's' description of the pain and fatigue involved was provided by the Scottish rider, Robert Millar, who won *le maillot à pois* (the jersey worn by the best climber) and came fourth in the 1984 Tour de France. Millar (*Guardian*, 31 July 1998) said:

> The riders reckon that a good Tour takes one year off your life, and when you finish in a bad state, they reckon three years …
>
> You can't describe to a normal person how tired you feel … In 1987, when I finished in a really bad way it took me until the end of November to recover; by that I mean until I could wake up and not feel tired as if I had already done a day's work.
>
> The fatigue starts to kick in on the Tour after 10 days if you're in good shape, and after five days if you're not in your best condition physically. Then it all just gets worse and worse, you don't sleep so much, so you don't recover as well from the day's racing, so you go into your reserves, you get more knackered, so you sleep less … It's simply a vicious circle.
>
> The best way of describing how you feel is that it's as if you were a normal person doing a hard day's work, you've got flu, and you can just about drive home and fall into bed. By the end of the Tour, you need sleeping tablets.

> You can't divide the mental and the physical suffering; you tend to let go mentally before you crack physically …
>
> Riding up one of the mountains in the Tour if you're feeling bad is like being sick. Physically, your body has a limit every day, there's only a set speed you can go at and it might not always be good enough.
>
> The pain in your legs is not the kind of pain you get when you cut yourself, it's fatigue, and it's self-imposed …
>
> It takes two weeks to recover from a good Tour, three months to recover from a bad one.

Given these physical demands, one can perhaps empathise with Millar's comment that 'I can understand guys being tempted to use drugs in the Tour'.

In 2001, a medical consultant who was working at that time with Lance Armstrong's US Postal Service team was reported as telling a medical conference in Spain that long stage races like the Tour de France 'are killing riders'. Luis Barrios, who had formerly worked with Tour de France winners Pedro Delgado and Miguel Indurain, also told the conference that the use of banned substances would be less damaging than the rigours of a day in the mountains: 'One stage of the Pyrenees will do far more damage to a cyclist's health than a therapeutic dose of certain banned substances' (*Cycling Weekly*, 15 December 2001).

Almost all of the media coverage of the doping scandal in the 1998 Tour de France was, perhaps unsurprisingly, heavily emotive and did little to enhance our understanding of the processes involved. One of the few exceptions, and one which brought out particularly clearly the relationship between exhaustion and drug use and the involvement of team doctors in this process, was a perceptive piece written in *The Times* (25 July 1998) by James Waddington. Waddington pointed to the enormous physical demands which the Tour makes upon riders; he described the Tour as 'not just healthy exercise' but 'close to physical abuse', and suggested that, in the attempt to keep their team members in the race, team doctors will draw upon an exhaustive knowledge of a range of substances – nutritional, hormonal and anabolic. He continued:

> It is a complex regime, with maybe 20 different components … Only the team doctor has this exhaustive knowledge, and thus the average professional cyclist with no scientific background becomes not a partner but a patient. He opens his mouth, holds out his arm, and trusts. That trust, not the reflex shriek of 'drugs, the excrement of Satan', should be the critical point in the whole discussion'.

Waddington's article makes two important points. The first of these is that, as he correctly notes, the 'reflex shriek of "drugs, the excrement of Satan"' is singularly unhelpful. His comments in this regard are very much in line with the argument about involvement and detachment made in the opening chapter of this book. The second point – and this is of course the central theme of this book – is that if we wish to understand doping in sport it is crucial that we understand the centrality of the relationship between elite-level athletes and practitioners of sports medicine.

Conclusion

In this chapter, we have sought to document the changing relationships between sports physicians and cyclists in professional cycling from the second half of the twentieth century and into the early years of the twenty-first century. We have shown how changes in the structure of professional cycling in the 1980s led to an increase in the size and complexity of teams, with the increasing employment of sports physicians and other sport scientists in professional teams and the increasing reliance of riders on sports physicians for all aspects of their science-based training and racing programmes. One aspect of these programmes, as we have seen, was the systematic incorporation of drugs into these programmes.

Christophe Bassons (2000), who was a non-doper (possibly the only non-doper?) in the 1998 Festina team, and Antoine Vayer (in Martel and Watbled, 2005), a former physical trainer of the team prior to the scandal, have suggested that the widespread use of doping revealed in the 1998 Tour de France reflected what they describe as the 'empiricism' among professional cyclists and their poor understanding of science. In this chapter we have argued exactly the opposite: that the systematic and organised use of drugs within cycling from the 1980s can be seen as an integral part of the rationalisation of cycling, a central aspect of which was the systematic application of medicine and science to training and racing. Far from being based on empiricism, the increasingly systematic use of drugs from the mid-1980s reflected the growing involvement of sports physicians in the supply, control and monitoring of drug use, and the systematic incorporation of drugs in increasingly science-based training and racing programmes.

References

Bassons, C. (2000), *Positif*, Paris, Stock.

Bastide, R. (1970), *Doping. Les Suhommes du Vélo*, Paris, Solar.

Brewer, D. B. (2002), Commercialization in professional cycling 1950–2001: institutional transformations and the rationalization of 'doping', *Sociology of Sport Journal*, 19, 276–301.

Brissonneau, C. (2000), À chaque sport sa formule magique, in F. Siri (ed.), *La fièvre du dopage. Du corps du sportif à l'âme du sport.*, ed. Autremont, Vol. 197, Paris, 109–119.

Brissonneau, C. (2007), Le dopage dans le cyclisme professionnel au milieu des années 1990: une reconstruction des valeurs sportives, *Déviance et Société*, 2, 129–148.

Brissonneau, C. (2015), The 1998 Tour de France: Festina, from scandal to an affair in cycling, in V. Møller, I. Waddington and J. Hoberman (eds), *Routledge Handbook of Drugs and Sport*, London, Routledge, 191–192.

Dubin, The Hon Charles L. (1990), *Commission of Inquiry into the Use of Drugs and Banned Practices Intended to Increase Athletic Performance*, Ottawa, Canadian Government Publishing Centre.

Fincoeur, B. (2016), *Le marché du dopage dans le cyclisme sur route belge et français: analyse de la demande, de l'offre et de l'impact de la lutte antidopage*, Unpublished PhD thesis, KU Leuven.

Hamilton, T. and Coyle, D. (2012), *The Secret Race*, London, Bantam Press.

Lagrue, P. (2004), *Le Tour de France. Reflet de l'histoire et de la société*, Paris, L'Harmattan.

Londres, A. (1999 [1924]), Devil's Island and the Tour de France, A cycle sport production, *Cycle Sport*, August 1999.

Louy, X. (2007), *Sauvons le Tour!,* Paris, Prolongations.
Marchand, J. (1963), *Le Cyclisme*, Paris, La table ronde.
Martel, L. and Watbled, R. (2005), Antoine Vayer sort du bois, *Entretien*, 12 December 2005. http://velochronique.jimdofree.com/2005/11/28/antoine-vayer-sort-du-bois-entretien (accessed 26 July 2023).
Mignon, P. (2003), The Tour de France and the doping issue, in H. Dauncy and G. Hare (eds), *The Tour de France 1903–2003*, London, Cass, 227–245.
Moston, S. and Engelberg, T. (2017), *Detecting Doping in Sport*, London, Routledge.
Paoli, L. (2019), The peculiarities of the role of the market for doping products and the role of academic physicians, in B. Fincoeur, J. Gleaves and F. Ohl (eds), *Doping in Cycling: Interdisciplinary Perspectives*, London, Routledge, 79–96.
United States Anti-Doping Agency (USADA) (2012), *Reasoned Decision of the United States Anti-Doping Agency on Disqualification and Ineligibility*, Colorado Springs, USADA.
Vincent, K. (1976), La F.F.C. frappe à nouveau, *Le Figaro*, 19 November.
Waddington, I. (2000), *Sport, Health and Drugs*, London, Spon.
Waddington, I. (2019), Changing patterns of drug use in professional cycling: implications for anti-doping policy, in B. Fincoeur, J. Gleaves and F. Ohl (eds), *Doping in Cycling: Interdisciplinary Perspectives*, London, Routledge, 31–44.
Waddington, I. and Møller, V. (2019), WADA at twenty: old problems and old solutions? *International Journal of Sport Policy and Politics*, 11 (2), 219–231.
Waddington, I. and Smith, A. (2009), *An Introduction to Drugs in Sport: Addicted to Winning?* London, Routledge.

Part 4

Sports medicine and the rediscovery of public health

11 Sport for all policy, sports medicine and public health

As we saw in Chapter 6, in the years after the Second World War sports physicians began to articulate, for the first time, a coherent professional ideology which defined the distinctive nature of sports medicine as a branch of practice. The distinctiveness of sports medicine, it was held, lay not in the specific illnesses or injuries experienced by athletes, nor in any special treatments which sports physicians were able to offer. Rather, the distinctive nature of sports medicine was held to lie in the specific nature of the body of the patient, for the body of the trained athlete – for so long regarded as a normal body – was redefined as 'special' or 'abnormal', that is it was held to be qualitatively different, both physiologically and psychologically, from the body of what was then called 'the man in the street', the 'normal' person, the non-athlete.

This redefinition of the body of the trained athlete as 'special' provided, as we saw earlier, a clear basis for the institutionalisation of the role of the sports physician as an essential part of the support team for elite athletes. But it also had a number of other consequences, one of which was that it pushed the practice of sports medicine even further away from its eighteenth-century origins in public health. If the focus of sports medicine was the abnormal bodies of trained athletes, and if the athletic body was distinctively different from the bodies of normal people then, by definition, it could have little to say about the bodies of 'ordinary' people, in much the same way that a paediatrician would have little to say about the bodies of geriatric patients. Malcolm (2017: 48) has correctly noted that any claim which the British Association for Sports Medicine (BASM) might have had to specialist status 'was far more oriented to performance than public health matters' (Malcolm, 2017: 48). The same was true of the work of other newly emerging specialist organisations in this area, such as the British Olympic Association's Medical Committee, established in 1959, and the Institute of Sports Medicine, established in 1963. Heggie (2011: 104) has noted that the work of these organisations reflected the changed nature of the athletic body at this time, for interest 'in general fitness, in physical education, in the "health of the nation" was stripped away, leaving a clear concentration on the elite, ab- or super-normal athletic body'. And no less significantly, the three issues which dominated sports medicine on an international level at this time were doping tests, gender tests and the effects of altitude on athletic performance, an issue which was of particular concern in relation

DOI: 10.4324/9781003563921-16

to the 1968 Mexico Olympic Games (Heggie, 2011: 105). It is difficult to imagine a research agenda further removed from public health.

However, beginning from the 1970s, and accelerating from the 1990s, sports medicine as a branch of practice began to rediscover its early origins in public health. How and why this process developed is the theme of this chapter. The central focus of this chapter is the UK, but a broadly similar process took place in most western countries.

Sports medicine and the rediscovery of public health

Before we examine the processes involved in this 'rediscovery' of public health, it is important to note that the growing interest in public health issues in the latter decades of the twentieth century did not diminish, and most certainly did not replace, the longstanding interest of sports physicians in elite competitive sport and in performance enhancement. Nor, significantly, did it reduce the involvement of sports physicians in doping; indeed, almost all the major case studies of medical involvement in doping documented in previous chapters took place in the 1980s, 1990s and the first two decades of the twenty-first century, that is to say during the very period when sports medicine practitioners were beginning to take an interest in public health issues. Thus the growth of interest in public health did not replace, but took place alongside, the continuing central interest of sports physicians in elite competitive sport and in performance enhancement, as well as the continuing involvement of sports physicians in the doping of athletes.

The second point to note is that the growing recognition of public health issues within sports medicine took place not because sports physicians were proactive in making the connection between sports medicine and public health but, rather, as a result of the way in which the actions of practitioners of sports medicine were constrained by the actions and policies of other key groups. The key policies in this regard were 'Sport for All' policies and similar policies designed to encourage more people to become physically active, and the key organisations involved in this process were the state, the physical education profession and the sports lobby.

The state

Within Britain sport has never been formally considered as part of the welfare state. However, some writers have suggested that, since the 1970s, sport has been elevated to near equivalence with the constituent elements of the welfare state. Coalter has noted that from the 1970s one can identify the development of what might be called 'recreational welfare', with a 1975 government White Paper, *Sport and Recreation*, defining recreational facilities as 'part of the general fabric of the social services' (cited in Coalter, 2007: 10).

Since that time, those who have argued for governmental support for sports development have sought to locate their arguments within the context of the contribution which, it is claimed, sport can make to public welfare, broadly defined. The development of this policy of 'sport for good' (Coalter, 2007: 8–24) placed sport more centrally within the spectrum of social policy, largely because of the wider social benefits which, it was claimed, were associated with sporting participation.

The benefits which have most frequently been held to be associated with increased participation in sport are undoubtedly those associated with improved health. However, there is a lengthy list of other claimed external benefits from sporting participation, including reducing social exclusion and breaking down barriers of class, ethnicity and gender; reducing crime, delinquency and drug use among young people; fostering community integration and renewal; fostering national identity and prestige; and personal development through benefits such as developing tolerance, cooperation, respect, trustworthiness and the development of social skills (Waddington, 2020).

Although it is not a central concern in the present context, it might be noted that there is little evidence to support most of these claims. For example, there is little evidence that sport, crime and drug prevention schemes are effective in reducing crime or drug use (Waddington and Smith, 2004; Nichols, 2007), while Coalter (2007: 172–173) has noted 'the limitations of much research evidence for the wider impacts of sport'. But for the moment we are not concerned here with the limited effectiveness of many of these policies. What is important is that, since the 1970s, successive governments in Britain (and elsewhere) have consistently adopted policies designed to encourage greater levels of public participation in sport and physical activity.

From the latter decades of the twentieth century, the promotion of physically active lifestyles has become a significant priority of much national, international and global policy in public health. The development of such policies may be regarded as part of the emergence of what has been called the 'new public health', a process which involved, from the latter years of the twentieth century, a shift in emphasis in health policy from cure to prevention (Nettleton, 2006: 234). The reasons for this change were fourfold: a growing recognition that increasing investment in medical technology had resulted in diminishing returns; a change in the pattern of disease, with a shift away from infectious diseases towards chronic diseases often related to social and behavioural processes; an ageing population which placed an increased stress on health services; and problems of coping with the cost of the seemingly infinite demand for health care. The financial problems associated with the increasing costs of healthcare have led to attempts, firstly, to control the supply side by making healthcare more efficient and, secondly, to control the demand side by encouraging people to modify their behaviour and to lead more healthy lives. The attempt to encourage people to adopt more active lifestyles may be seen as part of this latter policy.

Within Britain, this policy found expression in the latter part of the twentieth century in a variety of projects initiated by the government-funded Health Education Authority, such as *Moving On* (1995), *Promoting Physical Activity in Primary Care* (1996), *Young and Active?* (1998) and *Active for Life* (1998). Since then the Department of Health (2009, 2011) and Public Health England (2014) have regularly stressed the health benefits of physical activity.

Similar developments have taken place in other countries. In the United States, for example, the Surgeon General's report, *Physical Activity and Health* (US Department of Health and Human Services, 1996:1), sought to encourage people to become more physically active, pointing out that 'people of all ages can improve the quality of their lives through a lifelong practice of moderate physical activity'. On the international level, the World Health Organisation (2010) similarly emphasised the health benefits of physical activity.

But those involved in government public health organisations were not the only ones seeking to promote greater levels of participation in physical activity, for this also became an increasingly important goal of the physical education profession.

Physical education

Writing in 1991, Colquhoun identified what he called an 'explosion' of interest which was taking place in the physical education profession in teaching health-related issues, an explosion which, he suggested, was indicated by a burgeoning number of professional articles and curriculum guides in several countries, especially Britain, Australia, Canada and the United States.

This was not an entirely new role for physical education, for during the inter-war period in Britain, *The Health of the School Child*, the annual report of the Chief Medical Officer of the Board of Education, regularly made reference to the importance of physical education for the health of school children. However, Kirk and Colquhoun (1989: 417) suggested that

> the recent re-emergence of health matters to occupy a place of central importance in school physical education marks a new moment in both the production of physical educators' views of their professional mission and in the production of a new health consciousness in society at large.

The central objective of this emerging ideology of health-based physical education (HBPE) was to instil in children a pattern of behaviour which involved regular physical activity which, it was hoped, would be carried into adult life.

Colquhoun and Kirk (1987) identified several processes which, they suggested, had influenced this re-orientation of physical education towards health-related issues, including a growing societal interest in health matters, the prevalence of heart disease and the spiralling costs of medical care. To this might be added the fact that, in the 1980s, there was considerable uncertainty among physical educators about the nature, purposes and status of physical education within schools. For example, Alderson and Crutchley (1990: 38) noted that there was 'no professional consensus regarding what being "physically educated" really means' nor 'how that state is best achieved'. Associated with this lack of clarity concerning the nature and objectives of physical education, there was also concern among physical educators about the relatively low status of their subject vis-à-vis what were often considered more 'academic' subjects. Significantly, the development of HBPE not only provided a clear definition of a socially valued core objective of physical education – the promotion of health – but also enabled those involved in physical education to draw upon the prestige associated with medicine and science to provide what they hoped would be a more secure and 'intellectual' basis for their subject.

The sports lobby

The Sports Council was established by Royal Charter in 1972 as an arms-length body of government, and much of its work in the 1980s involved working alongside local authorities in promoting sport in the community. For example in 1982 it published its strategic document, *Sport in the Community: the Next Ten Years*, which argued for the need to target recreationally disadvantaged groups such as women, the disabled, the elderly and ethnic minorities. Such strategies were almost invariably and explicitly linked with the welfare benefits which, it was claimed, would result from these policies. Thus in its key strategy document, *England, the Sporting Nation*, the English Sports Council (1997:3) claimed that:

> The benefits of sport are well rehearsed – national identity and prestige, community development, personal challenge, as well as economic and health benefits. Sport is a central element in the English way of life.

Sport for all, injuries and sports medicine

There was, then, in the UK from the 1970s a systematic campaign from successive governments, from the physical education profession and from the sports lobby, to encourage greater levels of public participation in sport. In this respect, Britain was not unique. Similar policies were followed, not only in the United States, but in many countries in Europe – in Italy, Germany, France, Spain, the Scandinavian countries and in Central and Eastern Europe – where people were encouraged to take part in sport and physical activity, largely for the variety of welfare benefits which, it was claimed, resulted from these schemes (Heinemann, 2003; Porro, Martelli and Testa, 2020). However, as Elias (1978) noted, the implementation of social policy is a complex process which almost invariably generates unplanned outcomes. In the case of Sport for All policies, the most important unplanned outcome – and one which had important consequences both for public health and for sports medicine – related to the incidence of sport-related injuries.

In numerous publications over many years, we have consistently argued that the relationship between sport and health is very problematic, not least because the health benefits which are undoubtedly associated with physical activity (Academy of Royal Medical Colleges, 2015) are largely offset by the very high risk of (sometimes serious) injuries in sport (Waddington, 2000, 2007, 2008, 2010, 2023; Waddington, Malcolm and Green, 1997; Waddington and Murphy, 1998, Waddington and Smith, 2018). In this sense it might be said that the successful implementation of schemes designed to encourage greater participation in sport was *inevitably* associated with an increase in sports injuries. How serious was this problem in health terms?

Most of us are probably familiar with newspaper coverage of the injuries of our sporting heroes and it is certainly the case that professional sport is 'a violent and hazardous work-place, replete with its own unique forms of "industrial disease"' (Young, 1993: 373); for example, the risk of injury in English professional football is no less than 1,000 times the risk of injury in other occupations normally considered high risk, such as construction and mining (Hawkins and Fuller, 1999). But while the injuries incurred by non-elite athletes in mass sport and exercise rarely arouse much public interest, they actually constitute a far more serious problem in public health terms.

Large-scale, national studies of sports injuries are rare, but a study carried out by Sheffield University Medical School for the Sports Council in 1991 provided a good indication of the size of the injury problem associated with mass participation in non-elite, grassroots-level sport. This was the largest and most comprehensive study of sports injuries in Britain and it estimated that there are, in England and Wales, 19.3 million incidents resulting in new injuries and a further 10.4 million incidents resulting in recurrent injuries, making a total of no fewer than 29.7 million sport-related injuries a year. Sprains and strains of the ankles, knees, legs and back and arms were the most common injuries, but approximately half of all incidents resulted in what were defined as 'non-trivial injuries which were potentially serious' (fractures, dislocations or any injury to the head or face) (Sports Council, 1991: 2). The direct treatment costs of new and recurrent injuries were estimated at £421m and sports injuries were the cause of up to 11.4 million days off work, resulting in lost production costs of £575m. The total annual cost of all sports injuries was estimated at £997m. [all costs at 1991 prices] (Sports Council, 1991: 29–31).

Other studies in the Netherlands (Reijnen and Velthuijsen,1989; Dekker et al., 2000), the United States (Hootman et al., 2002; Gilchrist et al., 2011), Scotland (Campbell and O'Driscoll, 1995; Nicol et al., 2011) and the European Union (Kisser and Bauer, 2012) have confirmed the very high level of injuries in grassroots sport. Given these data, it is perhaps not surprising that, as early as 1982, one text on sports injuries was subtitled 'The Unthwarted Epidemic' (Vinger and Hoerner, 1982).

But what effect did this epidemic of injuries have on the practice of sports medicine?

Redefining sports medicine

In order to understand the significance of injuries in recreational sport for the development of sports medicine, we need to revisit once more what came to be defined, in the years after the Second World War, as the distinguishing feature of sports medicine, namely the focus on the 'abnormal' bodies of elite athletes. We also need to revisit the explanatory principle, outlined in Chapter 1, that 'one of the major constraints operating on the producers of any product is the structure of the market for that product' (Waddington, 1984: 180). In that earlier chapter, that principle was used to explain some of the characteristics of eighteenth-century medicine but, in terms of the importance of the market, what was true of eighteenth-century medical practice was no less true of the practice of sports medicine in the late twentieth and early twenty-first centuries.

The claim that the body of the elite athlete was 'special' or 'abnormal' – in a word, that it was different from the body of a 'normal' person – provided, as we have seen, a clear rationale for the practice of sports medicine as a distinctive branch of medicine, as well as establishing the role of the sports physician as an essential member of the elite athlete's support team. But it also had another important consequence: it defined the market for sports medicine as a niche market with, by definition, a very limited pool of potential patients. For if the focus of sports medicine was the bodies of elite athletes and if, as was claimed, these bodies had little in common with the bodies of 'normal' people, then sports physicians had little to offer the rapidly expanding number of those who were injured in non-elite recreational sport or exercise. What was the size of this niche market for sports medicine among elite athletes?

It is difficult to arrive at a precise estimate of the number of elite/professional athletes in Britain in the final decades of the twentieth century. However, it is possible to arrive at an approximation. In the 1970s and 1980s, Britain normally sent between 250 and 350 athletes to the multi-sport summer Olympic Games and around 50 athletes to the Winter Olympics. There were, of course, many more elite athletes in the main professional team sports. By far the largest of these, in terms of the number of players was (and is) association football (soccer). Professional footballers have long been highly organised in the Professional Footballers Association (PFA) in which virtually all professional players were/are members and, at the turn of the last century the PFA had a total membership, from the 92 Premier League and Football League clubs and from a number of semi-professional non-league clubs, of approximately 2,800 (Waddington et al., 2005). It is difficult to obtain accurate figures for the number of elite/professional players from the two codes of rugby at that time, but in rugby league in the 1980–1981 season there were 31 professional clubs in the national league, 16 in the top division and 15 in the second division, so the total number of players would have been far fewer than the number of footballers in the 92 professional football league clubs. The same is true for the number of rugby union players, which of course remained formally an amateur sport until 1995. In 1984, rugby union moved towards a national league system with the creation of two national merit leagues for the top 24 clubs. Of the major national team sports, cricket probably had the fewest professional players (even today it currently has only about 400 professionals). Though one can do little more than arrive at a rough estimate, it seems likely that in the 1970s and 1980s there were no more than at best a few thousand elite/professional athletes in Britain. To provide a basis for comparison, a detailed long-term study of the workload in a general practice in south-east London from 1950 to 1985 indicates that in the early 1980s, the list size of the practice was approximately 8,500 (Fry and Dillane, 1986). In other words, the focus of sports medicine on the bodies of elite trained athletes meant that the *national* pool of potential patients was almost certainly less than the size of *just one general practice* list at the time. And this, it should be emphasised, was during a period when there was a huge potential market for the treatment of up to thirty million injuries a year. The mismatch between the huge and growing public demand from patients requiring treatment for sports injuries and the (almost non-existent) supply of treatment from sports physicians, could hardly have been more striking. This epidemic of sports injuries and the associated search for treatment created a number of problems and dilemmas for sports physicians and for the key organisation within sports medicine, BASM.

Of course many of those who were injured in recreational sport or exercise did seek medical treatment. The Sports Council data (1991: 19) indicate that 25 per cent of those who incurred a new sports injury and 31 per cent of those with a recurrent injury received treatment for their injuries, meaning that approximately eight million people each year received treatment for sports and exercise-related injuries. However very little of this care was provided by doctors who would have defined themselves as sports physicians or who were members of BASM. The main providers of care were family doctors, hospital Accident and Emergency departments, physiotherapists, 'other doctors', other professions allied to medicine and 'others' (who included 35 non-orthodox practitioners) (Sports Council, 1991: 19).

One response to the growing epidemic of sports injuries was the development of sports injuries clinics. However, this again created problems for practitioners of sports medicine. The early clinics were hospital-based and often run by surgeons, whereas the BASM membership was largely made up of general practitioners and other primary care practitioners. In addition, while there was a developing market in private sports injuries clinics in the 1970s, some of these were set up by people who were not recognised as experts by BASM, which led to demands for the establishment of some system by which 'qualified' sports medicine practitioners could be distinguished from 'quacks' (Heggie, 2011: 148). In relation to the allegation that so-called unqualified 'quacks' were sometimes providing care, it is interesting to note that the Sports Council's report (1991: 19) found that almost as much care was being provided by 'others', who included 'non-orthodox practitioners', as was being provided by physiotherapists.

There was too, another important new dimension of this situation. Throughout the second half of the twentieth century, there were relatively few positions for physicians to work with elite athletes, and most of these were filled on a voluntary, unpaid basis. For example, Donald Macleod noted that 'There never was any money in rugby', and he recalled that he was a consultant surgeon in 1983 when he accompanied the British Lions to New Zealand for a twelve-week tour as the team doctor. Not only was he unpaid, but he was also dependent on the goodwill of his employers, the South-east Scotland Regional Health Board, who allowed him to accumulate his holiday entitlement for that year, so that he was able to take six weeks as paid leave and the remaining six weeks as unpaid leave (Holloway, 2017a: 6). Even at the end of the twentieth century, and even in the wealthiest and most highly professionalised of sports, English professional football, many club doctors provided their services on a voluntary basis – some even subsidised the club by the provision of medical equipment – while others accepted rates of payment which they knew to be well below the British Medical Association recommended scale of fees (none of this applied to club physiotherapists, almost all of whom were full-time employees of the club. However, many of these 'physiotherapists' held only a relatively low level qualification in the management of injuries, offered by the Football Association, which was not recognised by the NHS. See Waddington, Roderick and Parker, 1999).

For much of the second half of the twentieth century, the limited number of positions in elite sport had generally been filled by experienced clinicians who, like Donald Macleod, already had established positions and secure incomes from general practice or from hospital practice, and who could afford to work with elite level athletes on an unpaid basis because of their personal interest in, or their love of, sport. But the epidemic of sports injuries, and the associated increasing demand for medical care from those who were injured in mass sport and leisure activities, began to open up from the 1970s a new possibility, and one that was perhaps particularly attractive to younger, less established practitioners: the possibility of the practice of sports medicine not merely out of interest or love for sport, but *as an occupation*, either within private sports injuries clinics, or within hospitals.

The response to this situation on the part of BASM and other institutions such as the Institute of Sports Medicine was, in the first instance, to provide, and to encourage the provision by other medical bodies and colleges, of specialised courses in sports medicine, which proliferated markedly in the 1970s and 1980s (Heggie, 2011: 155). It might be suggested that the introduction of these specialised courses represented, in effect, an implicit acceptance of, and a willingness to engage with, this rapidly developing mass market for the treatment of injuries. More particularly, it might be suggested that the introduction of these courses functioned to provide BASM with a degree of control over this newly developing market by two means. Firstly, offering specialist qualifications provided a clear means of differentiating between those who were, and those who were not, entitled to call themselves 'experts' in sports medicine and who were therefore appropriately qualified to work in that field. And secondly, it gave to those who held a relevant specialist qualification a competitive advantage in the market over those who did not.

But if the changing structure of the market was a major 'pull' factor – that is a key process which pulled BASM towards broadening the scope of its interest beyond just the bodies of elite athletes – there was also an important 'push' factor, that is a process which pushed BASM in the same direction. This related to the attempt to seek specialty status for sports medicine.

The provision of specialised courses, in addition to providing BASM and its members with a degree of market control, also underpinned later claims for specialty status for sports medicine. Such demands were rarely heard before the mid-1970s, though they became increasingly common from the 1980s. The achievement of specialty status has considerable advantages for the members of the group claiming that status: it enhances the status of a particular area of practice and constitutes a clear statement of the legitimacy of that branch of practice in the eyes of the wider profession, it opens up possibilities for postgraduate education and research (and access to research funding) and it opens up the possibility of more employment opportunities in the area, including the establishment of hospital-based consultancies.

However, the establishment of specialty status is a complex and difficult process, not least because it is likely to arouse opposition from other practitioners and from other sections of the profession and, in this sense, the campaign for specialty status is, like any other form of status rivalry, a political process (it will be recalled from Chapter 3 that the profession had a long history of intra-professional rivalries, disputes and conflicts).

There were numerous disagreements and conflicts within the profession over the nature and status of sports medicine. In 1980 an orthopaedic surgeon described sports medicine as a 'pseudospecialty', claiming that it was 'artificial' to group patients 'according to the origin of their injuries' (cited in Heggie, 2011: 169). Heggie (2011: 147) also notes that not all doctors were in agreement with the basic principle of sports medicine – that athletes were different and therefore required special treatment – with some suggesting that athletes were actually *less* deserving than other patients because sports injuries were regarded as self-inflicted. One of the pioneers of sports medicine in Britain, Peter Sperryn, has recalled the 'vindictive hostility' towards sports medicine, and also claimed that he had been rejected for jobs due to prejudice against sports medicine, while John Lloyd Parry similarly referred to 'the hostility of the medical establishment' towards sports medicine (Reynolds and Tansey, 2009, cited by Malcolm, 2017: 51).

It is clear that there was a good deal of opposition from within the profession to the claim to speciality status for sports medicine, both from individual practitioners and, more importantly, from other medical professional organisations. Within the politics of the campaign for specialty status, it was undoubtedly the latter which was of major importance. In 1995 a working group representing sports medicine organisations within the UK had lobbied the Royal Colleges for recognition as a specialty. However, the Academy of Medical Royal Colleges appears not to have been very sympathetic, perhaps because it 'considered sport as elitist' (Holloway, 2017b: 6). Significantly, however – and it is significant because the organisation concerned was involved in public health – support was offered from the College of Public Health, if – but only if – 'exercise for the public was included' (Holloway, 2017b: 6), that is to say only if there was an explicit shift away from an exclusive focus on elite sport towards exercise as a public health issue. The constraints imposed by other sections of the medical profession were clearly of major importance; as the website of BAS(E)M acknowledges, it 'was becoming clear that in the UK, sports medicine as a specialty was unlikely to gain adequate support by itself and that the addition of exercise medicine was essential!' (https://basem.co.uk/about/history accessed 16/07/2024). In the following year, at a dinner which has a celebrated place in the history of sports medicine in the UK, the Chair of the Conference of Medical Royal Colleges announced the establishment of a Board of Sport *and Exercise* Medicine. BASM responded by setting up a special group to consider the situation, and the official historian of BAS(E)M has noted that the 'increasing pressure to include exercise medicine alongside sports medicine resulted in BASM changing its name to the British Association of Sport *and Exercise* Medicine (BASEM)' in 1999 (Holloway, 2017b: 6). Sports medicine finally achieved formal recognition of specialty status in 2005, but only by accepting a growing involvement in issues involving sport, exercise and public health.

Sport and exercise medicine and public health

We noted earlier that in the later decades of the twentieth century, there were a number of public health campaigns, both in Britain and elsewhere, that sought to encourage higher levels of participation in sport and physical activity on the part of the general population. In the first two decades of the twenty-first century, these campaigns have grown both in number and in the frequency with which they have been launched, largely as a result of the same constraints – most notably the continued escalation of the costs of clinical medicine and the claim that physical activity and exercise offer a relatively inexpensive and effective form of preventive medicine. Malcolm (2017: 55–56) lists no fewer than nine such campaigns which were launched in the UK in the period between 2004 and 2015 by the Department of Health, other government departments, medical colleges and lobby groups such as ukactive. In addition, the twentieth century has also seen the rise of a rapidly developing Exercise is Medicine movement, which was launched in a joint initiative by the American College of Sports Medicine and the American Medical Association in 2007, and which held its inaugural World Congress in 2010, attended by delegates from over 60 countries (Malcolm, 2017: 87). Not only have these campaigns been keenly supported by the medical profession, but the rediscovery of public health by those in the new specialty of sport and exercise medicine is also, it seems, laying the foundations for the emergence of a new sub-subdiscipline within sport and exercise medicine: sport and exercise psychiatry (SEP), which is held to be appropriate not just for elite athletes but also for non-athletes within the general population (Burger et al., 2024).

The rediscovery of public health by sports and exercise medicine may be seen as a further extension of the medicalisation process, for while the development of sports medicine in the period after 1945 extended medical control over the preparation of a small number of elite athletes, the incorporation of exercise within the medical remit extended medical control over an everyday leisure activity in which millions of people regularly participate. Central to this process has been that sports medicine has – Malcolm suggests 'arguably for its own self-serving ends' – become 'increasingly complicit in the reproduction of ideas linking sport and health' (Malcolm, 2017: 12).

Ideas linking sport, exercise and health are of course widely accepted not just in the UK but across a wide range of modern societies (Waddington, 2000). This does not however mean that these ideas, or the involvement of sports medicine in the reproduction of these ideas, are unproblematic. There are at least three dimensions to this problem which require us to: (i) briefly revisit some issues relating to sports injuries; (ii) examine links between the sport-health ideology and the ideology of healthism and victim blaming; and (iii) examine the limited capacity of sport to generate improved levels of health and welfare because sport is itself deeply embedded in the very structure which generates poor health and welfare: social inequality.

Sports injuries revisited

We have already noted that studies in several countries have all confirmed the high level of injuries associated with mass participation in non-elite, grassroots-level sport. A brief reference to two other studies will serve to emphasise the seriousness of the public health issues raised by these studies.

Three years after the national study carried out for the Sports Council in 1991, which we outlined above, a team from Sheffield University (which included two of the three authors of the original 1991 study) carried out a second study to ascertain the direct healthcare costs and benefits associated with sport and exercise. The health benefits of exercise (such as avoidance of chronic illnesses such as cardiovascular disease and osteoporosis) were weighed against the costs of treatment of exercise-related injuries. It was found that, whereas there were clear economic benefits associated with exercise for adults aged 45 and over, for younger adults (aged 15–44), the costs avoided by the disease-prevention effects of exercise amounted to just 20 per cent of the medical costs of treating injuries resulting from participation in sport and exercise. The authors concluded, 'there are strong economic arguments in favour of exercise in adults aged 45 or over, but *not* in younger adults (Nicholl, Coleman and Brazier, 1994: 109, emphasis added). A Dutch study, which produced similar findings to those of Nicholl et al. noted that these findings contrast 'heavily with statements of people who use the supposed health effect of sport as an economic argument to promote sport' (Reijnen and Velthuijsen, 1989, cited in Nicholl, Coleman and Brazier, 1994).

It is also important to emphasise that many sports injuries are serious; one study carried out within the EU estimated that there are more deaths in the EU member states due to sports injuries (7000 per year) than to workplace accidents (6080) or homicides (5540) (Kisser and Bauer, 2012).

But how does one square the data from these (and many similar) studies with data from other studies which have documented the many health benefits associated with physical activity – benefits which have led the Academy of Medical Royal Colleges in Britain to describe physical activity as one of the 'best buys' in public health, with the Chair of the Academy suggesting that 'if physical activity were a drug it would be classed as a wonder drug' (AMRC, 2015: 2).

In order to resolve this apparent contradiction, it is necessary to differentiate between three related, but very different kinds of activity: sport, exercise and physical activity more generally (Waddington, 2000). Many people within the sport policy community, both inside and outside government (e.g. within Britain the Department for Culture, Media and Sport and Sport England), have sought to promote sport by pointing to the well-documented health benefits of physical activity. However, almost all of those studies which are cited to support the idea that sport is good for health refer *not* to sport, but to physical activity or exercise. But physical activity and sport are *not* the same thing. Physical activity or exercise might involve walking or cycling to work, dancing, working in the garden, walking the dog or walking upstairs instead of taking the elevator at work. None of these are sport.

Although some authors make no clear distinction between sport and physical activity in general, the usual practice among sociologists is to define sport as a particular type of physical and social activity, with its own distinctive characteristics. Moreover, there are good reasons for this. As Guttman (2004) has noted, England's General Household Survey classifies people as sports participants if they walk to the bakery or the greengrocer's shop and, in a comment with which few will disagree, he writes that 'this does not seem reasonable'.

Most sociological definitions of sport include the element of physical exertion as an essential component. The leading sports sociologist, Jay Coakley (2007: 6) defines sports as 'institutionalized competitive activities that involve rigorous physical exertion or the use of relatively complex physical skills by participants motivated by internal and external rewards'. These key elements of organisation (e.g. the existence of rules), competition and a relatively high level of physical exertion are central to the work of most authors in this area (Waddington and Smith, 2018).

There are several important differences between the social relations which characterise physical activity and exercise, on the one hand, and sport on the other, and these differences have important implications for the injury risks associated with the different types of physical activity. Firstly, one cannot play sport alone, since one needs an opponent. This means that, in the course of play in many sports, each player is required to engage in rapid acceleration and deceleration, and sharp twisting and turning movements in order to outwit one's opponent (e.g. soccer, rugby, hockey, tennis, cricket), all of which involve high risk of injury. The competitive element of sport also encourages players to 'give their all', to play as intensively as possible – thus enhancing the risk of injury – and also encourages players to 'play hurt', that is to continue playing through pain and injury with all the health risks this behaviour entails (Roderick, Waddington and Parker, 2000; Waddington, 2021). In addition it is important to remember that many sports – and not just the obvious combat sports – are mock battles in which aggression and the use of physical violence are central characteristics. In this context, many sports have, in present-day societies, become enclaves for the expression of physical violence in the form of violently aggressive 'body contact'; indeed, in the relatively highly pacified societies of the modern West, sport is for many people the *only* activity in which they are regularly involved in aggressive physical contact with others.

These characteristics of sport mean that while exercise and other forms of physical activity, such as walking the dog or gardening, are health enhancing and relatively safe, competitive sport is, by contrast, much more dangerous. A study of the 204 Korean athletes who competed at the 2016 Rio Olympic Games found that no fewer than 56.3 per cent sustained one or more injuries during the Games, with an injury incidence of 150.9 injuries per 100 athletes (Yoon et al., 2018). And the injury rate also varies substantially from one sport to another; at the local level, the highest risks are, unsurprisingly, associated with intensive contact sports such as rugby, football, martial arts, hockey and cricket, while the activities with the lowest risk of injury are the moderate, non-contact, rhythmic (and largely non-competitive) activities involved in 'keep fit' and swimming (Sports Council, 1991). As Hardman and Stensel (2009: 250) have noted, 'while the incidence of serious health problems among people who engage in physical activity at a moderate intensity in moderate amounts is very low, participation in vigorous exercise or sport can be hazardous'.

Studies of this kind suggest that, if a major goal of Sport for All and similar policies is to improve people's health, then perhaps those in the sport and health policy community – and of course this includes sports physicians – should pause for thought to reconsider the kind of activities such policies are designed to encourage. It is clear that while gentle or moderate and regular non-contact physical activity is beneficial for health, the health arguments in favour of participation in competitive sport are much less clear.

Given that they have to compete for public funds with many other organisations, it is not perhaps surprising that many people within the sporting policy community have, by uncritically conflating the concepts of physical activity and sport, sought to claim for sport health benefits which are associated with many forms of physical activity but whose relationship to competitive sport is more problematic. This tendency is evident in the British government's policy document *Sporting Future* (DCMS, 2015), which made no attempt to differentiate between sport and other physical activities. Indeed, the DCMS (2015: 27) noted that while there are 'currently distinctions between sport and wider physical activity … those who responded to the consultation [which informed the development of its policy] told us that these distinctions are unhelpful, outdated and irrelevant, so we are removing them'. Most respondents to the consultation process are likely to have been sports stakeholders for whom the conflation of sport and physical activity may have important advantages, for example in accessing public funding. However, the decision by politicians and sport policy-makers to remove the distinctions between sport and physical activity is intellectually dishonest, makes no sense on health grounds and provides a misleading basis for public policy.

Sports physicians have, arguably, a particular responsibility to disaggregate the different types of physical activity in terms of their very different health consequences. For the most part, however, this much-needed critical edge to public policies in the area of physical activity and health has not been forthcoming. One notable exception is a former editor of *The Physician and Sportsmedicine* who, in 2003, referred to 'the increased physical, financial and emotional costs of injuries resulting from sports' and to the 'growing body of evidence documenting the enormousness of the sports injury burden'. He added: 'exercise … clearly promotes health, but competitive sports often may not. We need to own up to that fact, and shape our practices to address it' (Matheson, 2003: 2). Two years later he returned to the same theme, suggesting that physicians should 'emphasize, for our patients' sake, the difference between sports and exercise. Sports value winning and dominating, while exercise favors health and enjoyment' (Matheson, 2005: 2).

The ideology of healthism and victim blaming

As public health campaigns have developed with a focus on promoting the role of regular physical activity in promoting health, so a number of sociological critiques of these campaigns have also developed (Malcolm, 2017: 56). One of the most forceful and radical of these critiques is that relating to the ideology of healthism and victim blaming.

This critique was initially developed by Colquhoun (1991) as a response to the development of health-based physical education (HBPE) in schools from the 1980s, the central objective of which was, as we noted earlier, to instil in children a pattern of behaviour which involved regular physical activity which, it was hoped, would be carried into adult life. Although written specifically as a critique of HBPE, Colquhoun's argument applies with equal force to other public health campaigns which focus on increasing levels of physical activity.

Drawing upon Crawford's (1980) concept of 'healthism', Colquhoun argued that HBPE – and we might add more recent public health campaigns – are premised upon and help to disseminate the idea that our health is largely under our own control. More specifically, any such campaign, 'by focusing on individual lifestyle as the major determinant of an individual's health … has therefore been severely restricted in its potential for emancipation, social justice, equality and social change' (Colquhoun, 1991: 6).

The ideology of healthism, it is argued, serves to focus attention on individual responsibility for our own health and, simultaneously, to divert attention away from wider social processes – for example poverty, poor housing, unemployment, industrial pollution, or the poor quality or lack of accessibility of health services – which may be associated with high levels of illness. By thus shifting responsibility for health away from manufacturers, governments and other powerful groups, the ideology of healthism diverts attention away from the key issues in the politics of health. As Crawford (1980: 368) noted, it perpetuates the misleading – or at best, greatly oversimplified idea – that we can, *as individuals*, control our own existence. Moreover, our assumed ability individually to control our lives gradually becomes transformed into a moral imperative to do so for, suggests Crawford, we live in an era of a new health consciousness where to be unhealthy has come to signify individual moral laxity. Thus slimness signifies not only good health but also self-discipline and moral responsibility, whereas fatness, in contrast, signifies idleness, emotional weakness and moral turpitude. In this sense our bodies, whether slim or obese, signify not merely our health status for they also become, quite literally, the embodiment of moral propriety or laxity. Within this context, those who fall ill are increasingly likely to be seen not as unfortunate and innocent victims of processes beyond their control but, rather, as people who, through their moral laxity and lack of self-discipline, have 'brought it on themselves'. The Victorian differentiation between the 'deserving' and 'undeserving ' poor is, in some respects, in the process of being replicated in the differentiation between the 'deserving' and 'undeserving' sick.

In this regard, it might be argued that physical activity and health campaigns, which have of course been supported by those within sports medicine, represent not so much campaigns in *public* health, but rather a movement *away from public provision* and towards the *individualisation* of responsibility for one's own health.

Can physical activity improve levels of health and welfare?

It is not possible adequately to understand the relationship between physical activity and health and welfare without an understanding of the central importance of a key intervening variable: social inequality. There is a long history of studies of the relationship between social class and health, from Engels' classic *The Condition of the Working Class in England*, first published in German in 1845, to more recent studies such as *Inequalities in Health* (The Black Report) (Black et al., 1980), *Class and Health* (Wilkinson, 1986), *The Health Divide* (Whitehead, 1987) and *The Health Gap* (Marmot, 2015). But the publication of *The Spirit Level: Why Equality Is Better for Everyone* by the epidemiologists Richard Wilkinson and Kate Pickett (2010) was a landmark in our understanding of the relationship between social inequality, health and welfare.

Research by sociologists, epidemiologists, educationalists and others has long indicated that social inequality is closely related to a variety of social problems, including illness and reduced life chances, educational underperformance and crime. But what gave *The Spirit Level* its landmark status was, firstly, the huge mass of data which the authors gathered on a variety of welfare issues and inequality in relatively affluent countries and, secondly, the way in which these data were theorised into a compelling argument about the relationship between inequality and health and welfare.

Wilkinson and Pickett compared data on inequality and welfare from a large number of relatively affluent societies, including fourteen member states of the European Union and several countries outside the European Union, among them Japan, Norway, Canada, Switzerland, Israel, New Zealand, Australia and the United States. As a measure of inequality they used the ratio of the income received by the top to the bottom 20 per cent of the population within each country, a measure which is provided independently by the United Nations. Among the most unequal societies were the United States, Portugal and the UK, in all of which the richest 20 per cent received between seven and ten times as much as the bottom 20 per cent. The least unequal societies were Japan and the Scandinavian countries Finland, Norway, Sweden and Denmark, in all of which the top 20 per cent receive around four times as much as the bottom 20 per cent (Wilkinson and Pickett, 2010: 15–17).

Wilkinson and Pickett also developed an Index of Health and Social Problems, based on an analysis of as many aspects of welfare for which there are reliable data; health indices included rates of mental illness (including drug and alcohol abuse), infant mortality, life expectancy, adult and child obesity, along with other indices of welfare including children's educational performance, teenage birth rates, homicide rates, rates of imprisonment, conflict between children (bullying, fighting, etc.), and social mobility rates (Wilkinson and Pickett, 2010: 19). Their consistent finding, in relation to all these dimensions of welfare, is that how a country scores on the Index of Health and Social Problems is *not* related to how wealthy the country is, as measured by average Gross National Income per head, but *it is strongly related to the degree of inequality within the society*. Thus less wealthy countries with a relatively equal distribution of income have higher levels of health and welfare and fewer social problems than countries which are richer but more unequal. For example, the United States is one of the richest but also one of the most unequal countries, and it has consistently poor scores for almost all dimensions of welfare, including the very worst scores in the study for infant mortality rates, obesity, rates of mental illness, teenage birth rates, homicide rates and rates of imprisonment. Other countries with very high levels of inequality also scored badly on the overall index of welfare, whether they were very wealthy (e.g. the UK) or among the less affluent of European countries (e.g. Portugal). By contrast, the countries which consistently exhibited the fewest social problems and the highest levels of welfare were the Scandinavian countries and Japan, which were also the countries with the most egalitarian patterns of income distribution. In summary, the data in *The Spirit Level* showed that people living in societies with bigger income gaps between rich and poor are – independently of the wealth of the countries – much more likely to suffer from a range of health and social problems than those living in more equal societies. In a follow-up study, *The Inner Level* (2018), Wilkinson and Pickett documented in copious detail the relationship between reduced levels of inequality within a society and lower levels of stress and better mental illness and mental wellbeing. But if there is a clear relationship between social inequality, health and welfare, what is the relationship between inequality and participation in sport/physical activity?

In the UK, social class differentials in participation have changed little over the last 30 years. Data from 1990 indicate that 79 per cent of professional workers and 71 per cent of managerial workers had participated in at least one activity in the previous four weeks, compared with 55 per cent of semi-skilled and 46 per cent of unskilled manual workers (Sports Council, 1994). A study by the Department for Culture Media and Sport (DCMS, 2011) found that 63.7 per cent of those in professional or managerial occupations participated in sport compared with 42.3 per cent for those in semi-routine jobs. Data from Sport England (2019a) indicate that large class differentials remain. Seventy-two per cent of those in professional and managerial occupations took part in sufficient sport/physical activity to be classified as 'active' compared with 54 per cent of those in routine or semi-routine work and, significantly, the latter (33 per cent) were twice as likely as the former (16 per cent) to be classified as 'inactive'.

Moreover, just as specific sports have their own sex profile, so each sport has its class label. Coalter (2013) has noted that, in a study in Scotland, of the 30 sports for which robust data were available, the two lowest social classes were under-represented, in relation to their proportion of the population, in 28 of the sports, the exceptions being fishing/angling and snooker/billiards/pool. By contrast, the two highest classes were over-represented in 22 sports, proportionately represented in seven and under-represented in just one – fishing/angling. These class labels serve as a useful reminder that those who take part in sport and physical activities do so within the context of a wider society in which social class divisions remain important, and that the dynamics of class relations continue to privilege some groups and disadvantage others in the context of sporting activity. It might be noted that women and members of non-white ethnic communities are also under-represented in participation in sport and physical activities.

But how do these data feed into the discussion about the relationship between sport/physical activity and health and welfare? Perhaps the first point to note is that, if there are benefits associated with sport, it is clear that these benefits can only be generated insofar as people actually participate in sport. It is within this context that the above data on participation need to be considered. What, then, do these data tell us about the relationship between sport/physical activity, health and welfare?

What is clear is that the complex network of interdependency ties centred on class (and also on gender and ethic relations) locates people in relatively advantaged or disadvantaged positions, and that these positions of relative advantage and disadvantage relate to many areas of social life, including participation in physical activity and sport. The British data suggest that, though there are specific exceptions (e.g. black and ethnic minority people are more likely than white people to play cricket and basketball; see DCMS, 2011: 22), in general, people in these disadvantaged groups – the working class, women and ethnic minorities – experience in relation to sport and physical activity the same kind of limited access that they experience in relation to income, employment, housing and other goods and services. Commenting on the data from the Sport England survey, the chief executive Tim Hollingsworth noted that 'stubborn inequalities remain' and he argued: 'It isn't right or fair that people on a low income, women and black and South Asian people are still less likely to be active' (Sport England, 2019b). Opportunities to participate in sport and physical activity within Britain remain unequally distributed and in this respect it might be argued that the organisation of sport mirrors, rather than challenges, patterns of inequality within the wider society.

In this regard, the relationship between sport and physical activity on the one hand, and health and welfare on the other, is problematic, for two reasons. Firstly, insofar as there are health benefits to be gained from physical activity, these benefits are likely to be relatively limited in terms of their impact on national morbidity/mortality data. This is because, given the class-based patterns of participation in physical activity, any health benefits of physical activity will go largely to groups who, by virtue of their position within the social class structure, already enjoy relatively good health; much larger improvements in the national morbidity/mortality data would be achieved by improving the health of those in the lower social classes, whose health is much worse and therefore offers much greater scope for improvement. Secondly – and this is closely related to the first point – it is clear that the class-based patterns of participation in physical activity are likely to increase, rather than decrease, the class-based inequalities in health in the wider society.

It may be appropriate to conclude by locating this discussion within the context of the analysis set out in *The Spirit Level*. As we saw earlier, Wilkinson and Pickett (2010) provide a plethora of data indicating that levels of health and welfare are strongly associated with the degree of inequality within a society. If this analysis is correct then it has important implications for sport; as Coalter (2013: 16–18) has noted, 'it points to fundamental limitations on the ability of sports policy interventions … to address social issues in any meaningful way' for the analysis in *The Spirit Level* suggests that health and social problems 'are the price to be paid for such extreme and increasing levels of inequalities'. Moreover, even if sport does provide some degree of amelioration for some of these problems, this is likely to be very limited for, as Wilkinson and Pickett point out (2010: 26), 'our societies are endlessly re-creating these problems in each new generation'.

Finally, and in the context of the analysis by Wilkinson and Pickett, it should be noted that an analysis of income distribution in the UK from 1961 to 2015 noted that from 1977 until 1991 there was a long sustained period of continually rising income inequality, with a further increase in income inequality between 1996 and 2009, in which year income inequality was higher than at any time since 1961 (Institute for Fiscal Studies, 2019). Given this degree of inequality, it is reasonable to suggest that the relationship between sport, health and welfare is problematic and that one should not perhaps realistically expect that sport can make a significant contribution to improving health and welfare in Britain.

References

Academy of Medical Royal Colleges (2015), *Exercise: the Miracle Cure and the Role of the Doctor in Promoting It*, London, Academy of Royal Medical Colleges.

Alderson, J. and Crutchley, D. (1990), Physical education and the national curriculum, in N. Armstrong (ed.), *New Directions in Physical Education*, Champaign, IL, Human Kinetics, 37–62.

Black, D., Morris J., Smith, C. and Townsend, P. (1980), *Inequalities in Health: Report of a Working Party*, London, Department of Heath and Social Security.

Burger, J. W., Mafuze, B., Brooker, J. and Patricios, J. S. (2024), Championing mental health: sport and exercise psychiatry for low- and middle-income countries using a model from South Africa, *British Journal of Sports Medicine*, 58 (10), 519–521.

Campbell, H. and O'Driscoll, S. (1995), The epidemiology of leisure accidents in Scotland, *Health Bulletin*, 53, 280–293.

Coakley, J. (2007), *Sports in Society: Issues and Controversies*, 10th ed., Boston, McGraw Hill.

Coalter, F. (2007), *A Wider Role for Sport: Who's Keeping the Score?* London, Routledge.

Coalter, F. (2013), 'Game Plan' and 'The Spirit Level': the class ceiling and the limits of sports spolicy, *International Journal of Sport Policy and Politics*, 5 n(1), 3–19.

Colquhoun, D. (1991), Health based physical education, the ideology of healthism and victim blaming, *Physical Education Review*, 14 (910), 5–13.

Colquhoun, D. and Kirk, D. (1987), Investigating the problematic relationship between health and physical education: an Australian study, *Physical Education Review*, 10 (2), 100–109.

Crawford, R. (1980), Healthism and the medicalization of everyday life, *International Journal of Health Services*, 10 (3), 365–389.

Dekker, R., Kingma, J., Groothoff, J., Eisma, W. and Ten Duis, H. (2000), Measurement of severity of sports injuries: an epidemiological study, *Clinical Rehabilitation*, 14, 651–656.

Department for Culture, Media and Sport (DCMS) (2011), *Adult Participation in Sport*, London, DCMS.

Department for Culture, Media and Sport (DCMS) (2015), *Sporting Future*, London, DCMS.

Department of Health (2009), *Be Active, Be Healthy. A Strategy to Get the Nation Moving*, London, Department of Health.

Department of Health (2011), *Start Active, Stay Active: A Report on Physical Activity for Health from the Four Home Countries' Chief Medical Officers*, London, Department of Health.

Elias, N. (1978), *What is Sociology?*, London, Hutchinson.

English Sports Council (1997), *England, the Sporting Nation*, London, English Sports Council.

Fry, J. and Dillane, J. B. (1986), Workload in a general practice 1950–85, *Journal of the Royal College of General Practitioners*, September, 36 (290), 403–404.

Gilchrist, J., Thomas, K., Xu, L., McGuire, L., and Corondo, V. (2011), *Nonfatal Traumatic Brain Injuries Related to Sports and Recreational Activites among Persons Aged < 19 Years – United States, 2001–2009*, Washington, DC, Centers for Disease Control and Prevention, Mortality and Mortality, Weekly Report 60, 1337–1342.

Guttman, A. (2004), *'Rules of the Game', Sports: The First Five Millennia,* Amhurst, MA, University of Massachusetts Press.

Hardman, A. and Stensel, D. (2009), *Physical Activity and Health*, 2nd ed., London, Routledge.

Hawkins, R. D. and Fuller, C. W. (1999), A prospective epidemiological study of injuries in four English professional football clubs, *British Journal of Sports Medicine*, 33 (3), 196–203.

Heggie, V. (2011), *A History of British Sports Medicine*, Manchester, Manchester University Press.

Heinemann, K. (2003), *Sport and Policies: Six European Case Studies*, Schorndorf, Hofman.

Holloway, G. (2017a), A brief history of BASEM, Part 2, *BASEM Today*, 40, 6–9.

Holloway, G. (2017b), A brief history of BASEM, Part 3, *BASEM Today*, 41, 6–9.

Hootman, J. , Macera, C., Ainsworth, B., Addy, C., Martin, M. and Blair, S. (2002), Epidemiology of musculoskeletal injuries among sedentary and physically active adults, *Medicine and Science in Sport and Exercise*, 34, 838–844.

Institute for Fiscal Studies (2019), *Living Standards, Poverty and Inequality in the UK: 2019*, London, IFS.

Kirk, D. and Colquhoun, D. (1989), Healthism and physical education, *British Journal of Sociology of Education*, 10 (4), 17–-434.

Kisser, R. and Bauer, R. (2012), *The Burden of Sport injuries in the European Union. Research Report D2h of the Project 'Safety in Sports'*, Vienna, Austrian Safety Board.

Malcolm, D. (2017), *Sport, Medicine and Health,* London, Routledge.

Marmot, M. (2015), *The Health Gap*, London, Bloomsbury .

Matheson, G. (2003), Sports: hazardous to your health? *Physician and Sportsmedicine*, 31 (10), 2.

Matheson, G. (2005), Sports gone wild. Part 2: regaining proper perspective ? *Physician and Sportsmedicine*, 33 (3), 2.

Nettleton, S. (2006), *The Sociology of Health and Illness*, 2nd ed., Cambridge, Polity Press.

Nicholl, J. P., Coleman, P. and Brazier, J. E. (1994), Health and healthcare costs and benefits of exercise, *PharmacoEconomics*, 5 (2), 109–122.

Nichols, G. (2007), *Sport and Crime Reduction: The Role of Sports in Tackling Youth Crime*, London, Sports Council.

Nicol, A., Pollock, A., Kirkwood, G., Parekh, N. and Robson, J. (2011), Rugby union injuries in Scottish schools, *Journal of Public Health*, 33, 256–261.

Porro, N., Martelli, S. and Test, A. (eds.) (2020), *Sport, Welfare and Social Policy in the European Union*, London, Routledge.

Public Health England (2014), *Everybody Active, Every Day: An Evidence-based Approach to Physical Activity,* London, Public Health England.

Reijnen, J. and Velthuijsen, J.-W. (1989), Economic aspects of health through sport, Proceedings of an International Conference; Sport- an Economic Force in Europe, Lilleshall, UK, 20–22 November, 76–90.

Reynolds, L. A. and Tansey, E. M. (eds) (2009), *The Development of Sports Medicine in Twentieth Century Britain,* London, WellcomeTrust Centre.

Roderick, M., Waddington, I. and Parker, G. (2000), Playing hurt: managing injuries in English professional football, *International Review for the Sociology of Sport*, 35 (2), 165–180.

Sports Council (1991), *Injuries in Sport and Exercise*, London, Sports Council.

Sports Council (1994), *Trends in Sports Participation: Fact Sheet*, London, Sports Council.

Sport England (2019a), *Active Lives Adult Survey November 17/18 Report*, London, Sport England.

Sport Engalnd (2019b), Record numbers more physically active. https://www.sportengland.org/news-and-features/news/2019/april/11/record-numbers-of-people-in-england-are-getting-active/, accessed 19/8/2019

US Department of Health and Human Services (1996), *Physical Activity and Health: A Report of the Surgeon General, Executive Summary*, Washington, Department of Health and Human Services.

Vinger, P. E. and Hoerner, E. F. (eds.) (1982), *Sports Injuries: The Unthwarted Epidemic,* Littleton, MA, PSG Publishing Co. Inc.

Waddington, I. (1984), *The Medical Profession in the Industrial Revolution*, Dublin, Gill and Macmillan.

Waddington, I. (2000), *Sport, Health and Drugs*, London, Spon.

Waddington, I. (2007), Health and sport, in G. Ritzer (ed.), *The Blackwell Encyclopedia of Sociology*, Oxford, Blackwell, HE-LE., Vol. V, 2091–2095.

Waddington, I. (2008), Health, in D. Malcolm (ed.), *The Sage Dictionary of Sport Studies*, London, Sage, 127–129.

Waddington, I. (2010), Attavità fisica, m ovimento, sport e salute. Qual è il messaggio corretto per la salute publblica?, in S. Martelli and I. Waddington (eds.), *La Comunicazione per lo sport e la salute*, Milano, FrancoAngeli, 13–27.

Waddington, I. (2020), Sport and Welfare in Britain, in N. Porro, S. Martelli and A. Testa (eds), *Sport, Welfare and Social Policy in the European Union*, London, Routledge, 99–109.

Waddington, I. (2021), Researching pain and injury in sport, in E. C. J. Pike (ed.), *Research Handbook on Sports and Society*, Cheltenham, Edward Elgar, 321–336.

Waddington, I. (2023), From physically inactive to physically active: best practices for public health, in Y. Inoue (ed.), *Routledge Encyclopedia of Sport Studies*. https://doi.org/10.4324/9780367766924-RERSS64-1.

Waddington, I. Malcolm, D. and Green, K. (1997), Sport, health and physical education: a reconsideration, *European Physical Education Review*, 3 (2), 165–182.

Waddington, I. and Murphy, P. (1998), Sport for all: some public health policy issues and problems, *Critical Public Health*, 8 (3), 193–205.

Waddington, I., Roderick, M. and Parker, G. (1999), *Managing Injuries in Professional Football: A Study of the Roles of the Club Doctor and Physiotherapist*, Leicester, Centre for Research into Sport and Society, University of Leicester.

Waddington, I. and Smith, A. (2004), Using 'sport in the community' schemes to tackle crime and drug use among young people: some policy issues and problems, *European Physical Education Review*, 10 (3), 279–298.

Waddington, I., Malcolm, D., Roderick, M. and Naik, R. (2005), Drug use in English professional football, *British Journal of Sports Medicine*, 39, e18

Waddington I. and Smith, A. (2018), Physical activity, sport and health: what is the appropriate public health message? In G. Russo (ed.), *Charting the Wellness Society in Europe*, Milano, FrancoAngeli, 35–49.

Whitehead, M. (1987), *Inequalities in Health in the 1980s*, London, Health Education Council.
Wilkinson, R. G. (ed.) (1986), *Class and Health*, London, Tavistock.
Wilkinson, R. and Pickett, K. Williams (2010), *The Spirit Level: Why Equality is Better for Everyone,* London, Penguin Books.
World Health Organisation (2010), Global Recommendations on Physical Activity for Health, Geneva, WHO.
Yoon, J., Bae, M., Kang, H. and Kim, T. (2018), Descriptive epidemiology of sports injury and illness during the Rio 2016 Olympic Games: a prospective cohort study for Korean team, *International Journal of Sports Science and Coaching*. https://doi.org/10.1177/1747954118768686.
Young, K. (1993), Violence, risk and liability in male sports culture, *Sociology of Sport Journal,* 10, 373–396.

Part 5

Conclusion

12 Client control and the limits of professional autonomy – or why do doctors dope athletes?

In the previous chapter, we documented the rediscovery of public health by practitioners of sports medicine from the latter decades of the twentieth century and the early decades of the twenty-first century and we noted that in many countries sports medicine organisations are now actively involved in campaigns designed to encourage the general population to take part in what are held to be appropriate levels of physical activity. This process has constituted an important part of the recent development of sports medicine, not least because, as we have seen, greater involvement in the public health aspects of sport and exercise was seen within the medical profession more generally as a precondition for the recognition of sports medicine – or more precisely, sports *and exercise* medicine, as it became – as a specialist area of medical practice in the early years of this century. In this sense it might be said that it was precisely the long and close association between sports medicine and elite sport which constituted the major barrier to the recognition of sports medicine as a specialist area of practice, for many practitioners within the medical profession more generally did not consider that providing care for, and supervising the training programmes of, elite athletes constituted on their own an adequate basis for a 'proper' specialism.

But we also emphasised at the beginning of the previous chapter that the growing interest in public health issues from the latter decades of the twentieth century did not diminish, and most certainly did not replace, the longstanding interest of sports physicians in elite competitive sport and in performance enhancement. Nor, significantly, did it reduce the involvement of sports physicians in doping which had become increasingly apparent from the 1960s onwards; indeed, almost all the major case studies of medical involvement in doping documented in this book took place in the latter years of the twentieth century and the first two decades of the twenty-first century, that is to say during the very period when sports medicine practitioners were beginning to take an interest in public health issues. Thus the growth of interest in public health did not replace, but took place alongside, the continuing central interest of sports physicians in elite competitive sport and in performance enhancement, as well as the continuing involvement of sports physicians in the doping of athletes.

In the Introduction to this book, we noted that the involvement of sports physicians in the development, dissemination and use of performance enhancing substances and techniques has been conspicuously absent from histories of sports

DOI: 10.4324/9781003563921-18

medicine, particularly those which were written by 'insiders', that is by practising sports physicians. However, the relationship between sports medicine and the development and use of drugs in sport has occasionally been noted by others within the medical profession more generally. For example in 1988, *The Lancet* published an article with the title, *Sports Medicine – is there lack of control?* It suggested that although 'evidence of direct involvement of medical practitioners in the procurement and administration of hormones is lacking, their connivance with those who do so is obvious and their participation in blood doping is a matter of record'. It went on to conclude that:

> Members of the medical profession have long been concerned with the health and welfare of people in sport, but never have the stakes been so high. Evidence continues to grow that some are showing more interest in finding new ways of enhancing the performance of those in their charge than in their physical wellbeing. Surely steps must soon be taken to curb the activities of those few doctors practising on the fringe by bringing sports medicine beneath the umbrella of a recognised body within an accredited programme of professional training.
>
> (*Lancet*, 1988: 612)

With this comment, *The Lancet* was beginning to move towards a more adequate understanding of the relationship between sports medicine and the development and use of performance-enhancing drugs. In some major respects, however, *The Lancet* article failed to come to grips with important aspects of this relationship. In suggesting that 'evidence of direct involvement of medical practitioners … is lacking' and that that the search for new, and by implication, unethical, means of enhancing performance was confined to a 'few doctors practising on the fringe', *The Lancet* failed to grasp key aspects of the problem. Firstly, *The Lancet* appeared unaware of the growing body of data which, even at that date, indicated that there were more than 'a few' doctors involved in doping and that this was, at the level of elite sport, not uncommon practice. And secondly, they were for the most part not 'fringe' practitioners but, on the contrary, many of them, as we have seen, held prestigious positions within sports medicine at the national and even international levels. In this sense, what *The Lancet* saw as a problem concerning the lack of control of sports medicine was not a problem which was confined to the fringes but, on the contrary, one which went to the very heart of the practice of sports medicine in elite level sport.

In this respect, the publicly stated view of the British Medical Association (BMA) – not a body given to sensationalist statements – is perhaps more telling, because more accurate. In what was adopted as a BMA policy statement on doping in sport, the Association noted that 'it is clear that, at the elite level, the involvement of team doctors in doping is not uncommon and that it has not been confined to the former communist countries of eastern Europe' (BMA, 2002: 84). If it is the case that the involvement of doctors in doping is not uncommon – and we would suggest that the BMA's conclusion is supported by the abundance of evidence presented in earlier chapters – then we need to ask why this is the case. Why has medical involvement in doping in elite sport been a prominent feature in the development of sports medicine? In order to answer this question, we need to examine some other key aspects of the practice of sports medicine. It should be emphasised that the following analysis focuses on the practice of sports medicine in elite/professional sport, rather than the practice of those involved in public health or in the treatment of injuries among the general public.

Sports medicine: a very peculiar practice?

The sociological study of sports medicine is, relatively speaking, still in its infancy, although the number of published studies in this area has increased significantly since 2000 (Waddington, 2021). One of the early researchers in this area was Howard L. Nixon, who made an important contribution to our understanding of the sociology of risk, pain and injury in sport (Nixon 1992, 1993, 1994). Nixon's work focuses on the interrelationships within sports groups, or 'sportsnets' as he calls them, and attempts to identify the links between athletes and other members of the 'sportsnet', including other athletes, coaches and – and of particular relevance to us – team medical staff. Nixon suggests that a central characteristic of sporting culture is the 'culture of risk' and that the structural characteristics of 'sportsnets' expose athletes to what he called 'biased social support' – he refers to a 'conspiratorial alliance' involving sports physicians as well as coaches and administrators – that can influence and impose messages that foster the acceptance by athletes of risk, pain and injury and insulate them from, and inhibit them from seeking, medical care from outside the sport system. Walk (1997: 24) has suggested that one implication of Nixon's work is that 'medicine is practiced differently, more competently, and/or more ethically in nonsports contexts'. Although Safai (2003: 19) has suggested that in university sport, the 'culture of risk' is tempered by a concern for the health and safety of student athletes, there is abundant evidence, as we set out below, that in professional sport, clinicians are routinely constrained to deviate from established standards of good practice, both clinically and ethically.

These observations constitute the starting point for the following analysis, the central object of which is to consider whether there are aspects of the practice of sports medicine that might be considered as something less than what Walk calls 'proper medical care'. More specifically, we seek to examine whether the network of relationships in which sports physicians are involved limits their professional autonomy and constrains them to make medical compromises that their colleagues in other branches of medicine are less constrained to make. And if this is the case, is the not uncommon involvement of doctors in doping simply part of a more general process in which sports physicians are less constrained to behave in an ethical fashion than are their colleagues in other branches of medicine? It is important to emphasise that the following analysis does not focus on the individual characteristics of sports physicians – there is no suggestion that sports physicians are individually 'less moral' than their colleagues in other branches of medicine – but rather on the ways in which their actions may be constrained by their work situation.

Ethical issues in the practice of sports medicine in elite sport

Huizenga's book, *You're Okay, It's Just a Bruise* (1995), is a rare full-length exposé of the day-to-day life of a doctor in professional sport in the United States in the 1990s. Huizenga was a team physician to the Los Angeles Raiders and his book presents a revealing and disturbing picture of medical practice in the National Football League (NFL), which he describes as a system based on the 'dominating owner or coach selecting and paying the team doctor – who is then magically expected to have the player's best interest at heart' (Huizenga, 1995: 315). The owner's influence, he suggests, can be all pervasive and can impact on all aspects of the doctor's practice, including clinical decision-making. In this context, Huizenga documents the regular occurrence of malpractice and unethical behaviour by team physicians. Examples include the following:

1. The non-disclosure of information to players about their injuries and 'knowingly misrepresenting vital information to the patient' because the owner wanted the player to continue playing (pp. 258–271).
2. The prescription of anabolic steroids to 'bulk up' a player (pp. 149–150).
3. Doctors coaching young players to feign injury, against the rules of the NFL, so that they could deliberately fail an independent medical examination and thereby be placed on the injured reserve list. This allowed young players to develop their skills at the club while 'hiding' them from other clubs who might seek to sign them (pp. 140–142).

Huizenga also cites one other revealing practice. Under a collective bargaining agreement, the contract of a player could not be terminated while he was 'unable to perform the services required of him', that is while he is injured and Huizenga notes: 'Currently when a dispute arises, team orthopedists testify against the player – their patient. It's unheard of for a doctor in any other situation to testify against his own patient, unless that patient has literally committed murder' (p. 316). Huizenga concluded: 'It's not ethical for me to stay here. I can't be associated with this kind of medicine' (p. 125) and he eventually resigned in protest when the club owner supported a team doctor who deliberately withheld information from a player about a potentially serious spinal injury (pp. 266–267).

There have been few systematic empirical studies of what doctors in elite sport actually do on a day-to-day basis. Those empirical studies which have been done have mainly been carried out by sociologists, and they suggest that the unethical practices described by Huizenga were not confined to the NFL in the 1990s, for many similar practices have more recently been documented in other sports and in other countries. For example, a study of club medical staff in English professional football found that, as in the NFL, relevant information about their injuries may not be conveyed to players, or may even be deliberately withheld by doctors as a matter of club policy (Roderick et al., 2000: 175–176). Such practices clearly undermine any idea of informed consent by the player-as-patient in relation to return-to-play decisions.

With reference to return-to-play decisions more generally, Waddington (2006) found that club medical staff are often under a great deal of pressure, most notably from club managers/coaches, to agree to players returning to play before they are fit to do so and if the doctor refuses to agree, the medical advice against a return to play may simply be ignored by the coach/manager. In such situations, club medical staff appear to have two choices, both of which are problematic. They may simply adapt to and accept the situation, *in which case the quality of care they are able to offer is likely to be compromised to a greater or lesser degree*; in this regard, Hoberman (2012: 250) has suggested that the 'discounting or superficial treatment of athletes' injuries is the most common form of unprofessional sports-medial conduct'. Alternatively they may feel that their professional autonomy has been so circumscribed that they are unable to do their job in what they consider a properly professional manner. In the latter situation, they may choose to resign or, if they continue in the employment of the club, they are likely to find themselves in recurring conflict with the coach/manager, a situation which may be ended only when one or the other leaves the club.

A particularly striking example of the way in which team physicians may be constrained to make clinical compromises is provided by Malcolm's (2009) work on club doctors in English professional rugby. For a good many years there has been growing concern in rugby about the long-term consequences of concussion – one academic article described concussion as 'the hidden epidemic' (Marshall and Spencer, 2001) – and, as a response to this concern, the International Rugby Board (IRB) introduced a precautionary policy which required that any player sustaining a concussion should abstain from playing and training for a minimum period of three weeks 'and should only resume when declared symptom-free after a medical examination' (Malcolm, 2009: 196). One consequence of the IRB rule was that any diagnosis of concussion automatically deprived the club of the player's services. Malcolm noted that, within this situation, the resistance of players and coaches to a diagnosis of concussion led to 'a rejection of treatment protocols', the IRB guidelines and their underlying precautionary philosophy. Many doctors went to considerable lengths to avoid offering a diagnosis of concussion, with the loss of the player's services this would entail. Some doctors even argued that loss of consciousness – traditionally regarded in the medical literature as the most serious symptom of concussion – was on its own not sufficient to diagnose concussion (Malcolm, 2009: 202). Malcolm concluded that medical staff allow 'sporting performance criteria to override medical guidelines' (Malcolm, 2009: 191) and that a rule which was designed to protect players' health actually had 'the unintended consequence of leading clinicians to avoid the diagnosis of concussion'. He concluded that clinicians 'come to diagnose concussion in a way that they know will be acceptable to others' i.e. to players and coaches (Malcolm, 2009: 201). He describes that as a 'compromise', though one might suggest that rugby club doctors appear simply to have abandoned altogether a medical definition of concussion and to have substituted for it the lay understanding of coaches and players. As Malcolm notes, 'Allowing sporting performance criteria to override medical guidelines ... enables the diagnosis to become consistent with rugby players' (and coaches) own definitions of what constitutes an injury', thus allowing clinicians to 'minimize interpersonal conflicts' by replacing 'medically based diagnostic and treatment procedures ... by the understanding and definition of concussion dominant in the sport subculture' (Malcolm, 2009: 191). Clearly the professional autonomy of physicians is seriously undermined in a situation in which diagnosis and treatment come to depend on lay, rather than clinical, criteria.

There are, too, other studies which similarly suggest that the choice of treatment within the sports context may be heavily influenced by pressures from powerful lay people in the sportsnet. For example, there is evidence to suggest that club doctors in professional football may, because of the extreme pressures to return injured players to play as quickly as possible, be more likely than doctors in other, non-sport settings, to use what have been described as 'highly maverick biological therapies' (Faulkner et al., 2017: 136), a practice which, among other things, raises questions about the degree to which the practice of sports medicine is evidence based (McNamee et al., 2018). These 'maverick' therapies include the use of Traumeel and Actovegin and, most frequently, platelet-rich plasma (PRP). As McNamee and his colleagues note, there 'are serious problems with the quality of the evidence base for PRP' (McNamee et al., 2018: 349), which appears to be rarely used outside of the sports context. The evidence base for PRP across different injuries is 'inconsistent and uncertain' (McNamee et al., 2018: 350), while the National Institute for Health and Care Excellence (NICE), which has examined the use of PRP in the treatment of osteoarthritis of the knee (a common condition in [former] footballers), has concluded that the quality of evidence is too poor to support any verdict on PRP's effectiveness and, as a consequence, within the National Health Service, 'this procedure should only be used with special arrangements for clinical governance, consent and audit or research' (cited in NcNamee et al., 2018: 351).

However, the studies by Faulkner et al. (2017) and McNamee et al. (2018) indicate that the use of PRP is not unusual within professional football, even though most of the club doctors who took part in the study by McNamee et al. (2018: 355) 'were all well aware of the lack of robust evidence base for PRP'. Notwithstanding their general lack of confidence in the effectiveness of this treatment, club doctors felt constrained to use PRP because they were often under a great deal of pressure, particularly from players' agents, to do so. One experienced club doctor explained his actions by saying that, if he agrees to treat an injured player with PRP:

> it stops him going and getting a treatment from somewhere else because he hasn't been offered it by me. And I would rather control the degree of mismanagement.
>
> (McNamee et al., 2018: 355)

This doctor's choice of words – 'to control the degree of mismanagement' – clearly indicates the treatment compromise which he felt constrained to accept. It might be noted that it also bears similarities with the argument used in the 1960s by French sports physicians – that it is better (safer) that they controlled the doping process, rather than leave it to athletes themselves, or unqualified team *soigneurs*. It is also identical to the argument used by Dr Jamie Astaphan, who was the doctor who supplied drugs to Ben Johnson and numerous other athletes, to rationalise his involvement in doping. Astaphan told the Dubin Commission (Dubin, 1990: 251)

> The axiom among track and field plus other athletes was 'if you don't take it, you won't make it', so if I didn't monitor them and if I didn't give it to them, they were going to get it elsewhere ... They came to me for advice and for supervision, and I thought it was my responsibility to do this.

McNamee and his colleagues (2018: 344) also noted, in relation to the use of such unproven treatments, the use by clinicians of 'deceptive, placebo-like, practices ... that challenge dominant understandings of informed consent in medical ethics'.

There is also evidence that it is not unusual for ethical rules governing patient confidentiality to be breached in elite sport. The study of club medical staff in English professional football found that there was no commonly held understanding governing the management of confidential issues and that there were considerable variations from one club to another in terms of both the amount, and the kind, of personal information about players – for example information about players' drinking habits, or other aspects of their personal lifestyles – which medical staff passed on to coaches/managers (Waddington, Roderick and Parker, 1999; Waddington and Roderick, 2002). The authors documented serious breaches of medical confidentiality by club doctors and physiotherapists, which they described as a 'matter of serious concern'.

In a follow-up study, Waddington, Scott-Bell and Malcolm (2019: 659–660) found that club medical staff were still 'often under a great deal of pressure from managers to deviate from established standards of good [medical] practice', that staff are pressured to release potentially confidential information 'and that there were still considerable variations from one club to another in terms of the amount and kind of information about players that is communicated to the manager'.

The most significant change in relation to the management of confidentiality between the two studies was that, by the time of the second study, many clubs had responded to concerns about confidentiality by requiring players to sign a general confidentiality waiver (see also Anderson and Gerrard, 2005; Malcolm and Scott, 2014). These were mentioned by several interviewees, who seemed to see these as resolving the problem of confidentiality; one club doctor interviewee said: 'When they sign a contract to play for the club they ... sign to have released to the club any information that is important about their physical health and wellbeing... so they sign a consent form' (Waddington, Scott-Bell and Malcolm, 2019: 656). Malcolm and Scott (2014: 1412) similarly noted in their study of British Olympic Association (BOA) doctors that the use of such general waivers is relatively common, although they point out that 'the BOA's position statement on athlete confidentiality implies that consent should be specific, not reliant on open-ended or general permission, and the exception not the norm' and they suggest that general confidentiality waivers of this kind 'may contain elements of coercion'. Holm, McNamee and Pi Gozzi (2011) have similarly argued that consent to disclosure should be specific and the sports physician should not rely on any more general or open-ended consent given by the athlete patient (e.g. in an employment contract). Significantly, this is also the position of the Faculty of Occupational Medicine, which states that consent 'must be given freely, under no duress or threat, and applies only for the time and event for which it is given' (Faculty of Occupational Medicine, 1999: 3). Quite clearly, the requirement for players to sign a general confidentiality waiver when they sign a contract with a new club raises very obvious questions in relation to whether such consent can properly be regarded as 'freely given'.

A study of 16 sports physicians in New Zealand revealed a similar lack of consistency in dealing with confidential issues. Some had accepted contracts which actually obliged them to share medical information with coaches and team management, and five said they were prepared to disclose information, even against the wishes of the athlete, but in line with their contractual obligations. Ten physicians indicated they would keep such information confidential, citing a commitment to traditional obligations to confidentiality, while one practitioner was unsure of what s/he would do in these circumstances (Anderson, 2009).

It might be noted that the ethical guidelines in relation both to return-to-play decisions and medical confidentiality within sport are quite clear. In its handbook, *Medical Ethics Today*, the BMA (BMA, 2003: 596) referred to the findings of Waddington and Roderick (2002) on confidentiality and emphasised that:

> Ethically, sports doctors need to be aware that their chief loyalty is to their patients, and that, contractual obligations notwithstanding, the duty of medical confidentiality remains unchanged.

This also remains the advice to sports physicians from the Fédération Internationale de Médecine Sportive (FIMS), which states unambiguously that 'the physician's duty to the athlete must be his/her first concern and contractual and other responsibilities are of secondary importance' (FIMS, 2024). The UK General Medical Council (GMC) has similarly noted that 'patients have a right to expect that [doctors] will not disclose any personal information [...] unless they give permission' (GMC, 1995). However, it seems that elite sportspeople may not infrequently be denied a right which patients in other medical settings routinely enjoy.

The BMA also made reference to the work of Waddington, Roderick and Parker (1999) and Roderick, Waddington and Parker (2000) on return-to-play decisions, the provision of information to players and on 'playing hurt' – that is the constraints on players to continue playing through pain and injury – and it noted that players 'who have sustained injuries may come under pressure from managers to continue to play and that this 'may be the case even when continuing to play may exacerbate injuries or incur risk of long term damage'. It emphasised that:

> The doctor's chief obligation must be to the long term health and wellbeing of individual players. In such a situation, doctors must inform both the player and the manager of the risks involved so that both parties can make an informed decision about whether play should continue.
>
> (BMA, 2003: 596)

While the ethical guidelines are clear, the research evidence indicates that the day-to-practice of sports medicine in professional/elite sport by no means always complies with these guidelines. In addition to the problems associated with confidentiality issues and withholding information from players, mention might also be made of medical involvement in faking an injury – for example the infamous 'Bloodgate' incident in English rugby (Waddington, 2012) – and misusing clinicians' privileged access to injured players in the field of play to convey tactical information (Devitt and McCarthy, 2010). Anderson and Jackson's (2013) analysis of sports physicians in New Zealand similarly reveals expectations and pressures that compromise their professional standards, while other studies have highlighted clinicians' submission to the values of their more powerful clients such as coaches, managers and players (Scott and Malcolm, 2015).

In summary, the existing studies of day-to-day medical practice within professional/elite sport suggest that breaches of confidentiality are not unusual and, indeed, may even be commonplace; that it is by no means rare for information about their injuries to be withheld from players and that, on occasions, this may be done routinely as a matter of club policy; that club medical staff routinely make medical compromises in their diagnosis and treatment of players' injuries and that, in some cases, they may, in effect, simply abandon a medical understanding and substitute a lay understanding; and that doctors within sport may be subject to pressure to deviate from good medical practice in other ways described above. As Malcolm (2006a: 377) has noted, 'researchers have exposed numerous elements of poor medical practice in sport', and elsewhere he has suggested that the 'most enduring legacy of this body of [sociological] work is the "revelation" that medical care in sport simply did not function in accordance with the principles more generally accepted for this, or related, professions' (Malcolm, 2014: 28). More specifically, he has suggested that 'primary medical ethical principles such as confidentiality, privacy, patient autonomy and informed consent cannot be assumed to be operative in sports medicine' (Malcolm, 2017: 121). Given this situation it might be argued that much of the data generated by these studies suggest that one implication of Nixon's work on risk, pain and injury – that the nonsport world is, as Walk (1997: 24) puts it, 'more medically prudent that the sport world' – may have a good deal of substance.

If it is the case, as these data would seem to suggest, that doctors who practise in elite sport are subject to constraints which limit their professional autonomy more than is the case in other types of medical practice, how can we explain this?

Conflicts in the role of team doctor

The role of the club doctor in professional/elite sport is often likened to that of the 'family doctor', in which the relationship with the patient is normally underpinned by two fundamental assumptions:

1. The doctor's skill is used exclusively on behalf of the patient;
2. The doctor is not acting on behalf of anybody else whose interests may conflict with those of the patient.

However, this comparison is somewhat misleading, for these assumptions may not apply in the same way in the work situation of the doctor in elite sport. Of particular significance in this regard is that the team doctor 'provides medical services to athletes that are arranged for, or paid for, at least in part, by an institution or entity other than the patient' (Mitten, 2002: 8). Such an arrangement raises a series of potential problems for, as the BMA (2003: 595) has noted:

> Doctors who are employed by sports teams and by sports clubs may find themselves subject to the tension of conflicting loyalties. On the one hand, they are agents of the team or club with the contractual obligations of an employee, and, on the other, as doctors, they are advocates for the individual athletes or players who are their patients.

Clearly the club, which employs the doctor, has a legitimate interest in the health of players and in the management of their injuries. However, it has been noted that where medical staff are employed by the team management, 'this may lead to an explicit expectation on the part of management or coaching staff of loyalty to them ... [which] may not always be in the best interests of the athlete' (Roy and Irvin, 1983: 7). Crane, who was the Arsenal club doctor and also the doctor to the English national football team, has suggested that key aspects of the relationship between club doctor and player are *not* like those that apply in general practice, but rather those that apply to the relationship 'between an occupational physician and an employee of the company' and he notes that in this respect, the physician 'may be employed by the company primarily to serve its interest. *There may arise, therefore, a conflict of loyalties'* (emphasis added) (Crane, 1990: 332).

The comparison with the role of the occupational physician is in some respects helpful, not least because the focus on a potential conflict of loyalties goes some way towards helping us understand the structural conditions which are associated with what appear to be regular breaches of medical ethics in key areas of the practice of sports medicine. However, it is important to recognise that, whatever the nature of these potential conflicts of interest, the ethical guidelines of all the relevant medical organisations – the BMA, FIMS and the GMC – are all unambiguously clear on this issue: whatever contractual obligations a team doctor may have, these are of secondary importance and the first responsibility of doctors is to their individual players as patients (it might be noted that the Faculty of Occupational Medicine has similarly noted that the GMC has set out 'the general standards that the public have a right to expect of their doctors', that occupational physicians 'are required to work to these standards' and that the guidance published by the GMC 'applies to all doctors' (Faculty of Occupational Medicine, 1999: 5). It is important to emphasise that being a club doctor or team physician does *not* release the practitioner from the normal ethical responsibilities of doctors towards their patients.

But if the comparison with occupational physicians is helpful in understanding – though not, of course, in excusing – breaches of clinical and ethical standards, it can on its own provide only very partial answers, not least because there are some very important differences between the role of doctors in elite sport and the role of a doctor working in more conventional forms of occupational medicine.

Particularly important in this respect is the fact that while occupational physicians may be involved in the medical examination of individual workers from time to time, and will more generally be called on to advise on the nature and extent of work-related health risks to workers, to the environment or to the public, they are unlikely to have any strong personal identification with the product being produced by the company which employs them. We suggest that, in marked contrast, there is an abundance of evidence to indicate that a large majority of sports physicians working in professional/elite sport do strongly identify with – even have a passion for – the product produced by the sports organisations within which they work, and to which they themselves contribute – that is to say, the production of the elite level sporting performance. This leads us to suggest that elite-level sport must be understood as a unique work situation for medical practitioners, for it is not only very different from more conventional forms of occupational medicine but also from other forms of medical practice such as general practice (primary care) and hospital medicine. If we wish to develop our understanding of ethical breaches in sports medicine, and in particular what many people would perhaps consider the most serious breach of medical ethics – medical involvement in doping – then we need to develop a more detailed analysis of the unique work situation of sports physicians in elite sport.

Client control and medical practice

In *Profession of Medicine*, which is properly regarded as a classic in medical sociology, Freidson (1970: 88) noted that 'Deficient behavior on the part of a professional tends to be explained as a result of being a deficient kind of person, or at least of having been inadequately or improperly "socialized" or educated in professional school'. However, Freidson suggested that there was some 'very persuasive evidence', from a variety of studies of practising physicians and lawyers, which indicated that professional socialisation had only limited value in explaining some important elements of professional performance. More specifically, he argued that critical elements of professional behaviour – including the level of technical performance, the approach to the client, 'cynicism' and ethicality – do not vary so much with the individual practitioner's formal professional training as with the social setting within which they work after graduation (Freidson, 1970: 89–90). The key differentiation which Freidson made in this regard was between two polar types of medical practice: (i) colleague-dependent practice, in which interaction is primarily dependent on the professional evaluations and decisions of the doctor and their professional colleagues, and (ii) client-dependent practice, in which interaction between doctor and client is largely dependent on the lay evaluations and decisions of clients.

Central to understanding the position of practitioners of sports medicine in elite sport is that they are involved in a form of practice that is heavily client-dependent rather than colleague dependent, that is to say, interaction between doctor and client is largely premised on the lay culture, evaluations and decisions of clients rather than those of professional colleagues. Thus whereas the hospital-based doctor is surrounded by professional colleagues, is subject to their evaluation and is expected to be responsive to the clinical and ethical standards which they share, the physician who is contracted, for example, to a professional cycling team or football club is not surrounded by or subject to evaluation by professional colleagues but is much more subject to evaluation by, and is therefore much more dependent on, the lay demands of their clients, for it is they, rather than professional colleagues, who will judge the success or failure of the practice.

In this regard, the contrasts between the position of the hospital-based doctor and the team doctor are striking. Hospital doctors not only work in institutions which are major centres of professional power, where professional values emphasising health are uppermost and where lay influences are minimal, but they are also normally the most powerful occupational group within the hospital, enjoying high status within these institutional bastions of professional power and, as such, their authority and expertise are rarely challenged.

In marked contrast, the team doctor works within an organisation in which the key values are not professional values relating to health, but lay values relating to sporting success and, within this situation, sports medicine 'becomes a form of industrial medicine that values productivity over health' (Hoberman, 2002: 208). And if hospital doctors are the highest status workers – the 'stars', as it were – within the hospital, the 'stars' within sports clubs are those who are centrally involved in the pursuit of sporting success – the players and coaches – while the doctors are reduced to the role of lower status 'service workers', whose job it is to look after those on whom, it is held, the success of the club really depends. And while the authority and expertise of the hospital doctor are rarely questioned, the authority and expertise of the team doctor may, as in the case of club doctors in some professional team sports, be regularly challenged, rejected or simply ignored.

Significantly, their remuneration and status within the clubs is often consistent with their position as service workers. Huizenga, for example, records that he 'apologetically' raised the issue of his salary with the owner of the Los Angeles Raiders, who offered him, in a 'take it or leave it' manner, an annual salary which was less than many players received for a single game (Huizenga, 1995: 63). Waddington et al. found a similar situation in English professional football. The doctor at one Premier League club, who was nearing retirement, said that he was trying to move the club towards a situation in which his successor would be paid a proper professional salary and would have a clearly defined and recognised professional role within the club:

> They will be wanting a younger man, say within two years, but I would like … to get the club to a situation where there is a job description, precisely what the doctor does, there is a contract as well, fee paying is sorted out … so that this club will be taken to a level whereby they see this as a professional job.

The doctor added that 'I have trouble now, I send in my bill every year and they say, "Phew, you're charging us a lot, Doc", but really, it's peanuts' (Waddington, Roderick and Parker, 1999: 13–14).

Another club doctor indicated that he received just £5,200 per year for his services, even though he had calculated that, applying the BMA's recommended scale of charges to the number of hours he worked, he should have been receiving £25,000 (Waddington, Roderick and Parker, 1999: 9–10, 13–14). While doctors working for clubs in the higher divisions of English football were normally paid, all of them stressed that the pay was relatively modest and that the salary they received was not the main reason why they did the job. Few clubs offered rates of pay which doctors would normally expect to be paid for their professional services in other situations and, among lower division clubs, some doctors did not receive any payment; the doctor of one Third Division club explained that it was he who actually subsidised the club by providing some medicines and items of equipment from his own general practice surgery (Waddington, Roderick and Parker, 1999: 9–10).

Not only do club doctors work in a situation which is dominated by lay sporting values but this is also a situation in which, unlike doctors in many other settings, they are frequently professionally isolated. For example Malcolm (2006a: 383) noted that rugby club doctors 'tend to work in isolation from other professional colleagues', while a football club doctor whose advice against playing injured players was constantly ignored by the manager complained that his position was difficult because he was, as he put it, 'a single voice and if I disagreed with what was going on, then there were a lot more people around … to perhaps try to persuade me to change my mind' (Waddington, 2000: 77). Moreover, not only were club doctors professionally isolated within the club, but there were also relatively few opportunities for them to meet professionally with doctors from other clubs (Waddington, Roderick and Parker, 1999: 14). As Freidson has noted:

> All else being equal in this situation of minimal observability by colleagues and maximum dependence on the lay referral system, we should expect to find the least sensitivity to formal professional standards and the greatest sensitivity to the local lay standards.
>
> (Freidson, 1960: 381)

This is, it is suggested, what we frequently find in the case of sports medicine.

But the analysis above raises an obvious question. It has been suggested that the situation of medical practice in professional/elite sport is one which constrains sports physicians to orientate themselves primarily towards the demands of their lay clientele – which in this case consists of other members of the sportsnet, typically including the athletes themselves but also coaches/managers and, of increasing importance, players' agents – rather than towards the community of medical practitioners and that this in turn is likely to constrain practitioners to make both ethical and clinical compromises that they would not be required to make in other practice situations. But if club doctors are constrained to make such medical compromises, and also to accept what they would, in other circumstances, certainly regard as unacceptable rates of pay, then we need to ask: why do doctors accept such forms of employment? On this issue the evidence seems relatively clear cut.

Job motivation

In Chapter 5, we saw that there is a long history of the relationship between a passion for sport/playing sport and involvement in the practice of sports medicine and we noted that many key figures in the development of sports medicine in England, France and Germany had themselves been high level athletes. We also noted that Viaud's work (2009a, 2009b) indicates a continuing and strong relationship between sports physicians' personal participation in sport and their practice of sports medicine in modern France.

In the UK there is very direct evidence of the continuing importance of a passion for sport as the central motivation for involvement in the practice of sports medicine. In the study of club doctors in English professional football (Waddington, Roderick and Parker, 1999), it was found that by far the most common motivation which led doctors to accept employment as club doctors related not to professional goals, such as improving clinical expertise or qualifications, or moving into sports medicine as a full-time career – most club doctors continued to work in another area of medicine which provided their main source of income – but, rather, it derives from their longstanding love of sport and, in some cases, their commitment to a particular team. One club doctor, whose father had been the previous club doctor and who had been a fan of the club for many years, explained: 'I would find it difficult to imagine why anybody would want to do it if they weren't a fan. I mean it's not very well paid'. This doctor added: 'I did medicine so that I could be the team doctor – I wasn't interested in any other team'. Another club doctor said: 'Basically although I'm 46 there is a ten year old boy inside saying "Fantastic! Fantastic!"', while another doctor said that he did the job as he had always enjoyed playing football and being a club doctor was 'the next best thing to playing' (Waddington, Roderick and Parker, 1999: 10). Similarly, in a study of English professional rugby union, Malcolm (2006b: 170) noted that the most commonly cited motivations for acting as club doctor were 'support for the team' (82.4 per cent) and a 'general interest in sport' (67.6 per cent) with just 5.5 per cent indicating that their professional interest in sports medicine was a major motivational factor. Within rugby, the centrality of practical sporting experience as an aspect of the occupational culture of sports medicine was very clearly brought out in an essay by Ken Kennedy, a sports physician and former rugby player, in which he listed what he considered the ideal qualities of the rugby club doctor. These included knowledge of traumatology and the kinesiology of rugby, rehabilitation and orthopaedics and good referral contacts but, significantly, he adds that '*most importantly* the doctor should have an affinity for the game and the people in it' (Kennedy, 1990: 315, emphasis added).

In the American context, Huizenga describes a visit to the office of Dr Rosenfeld, who was a senior doctor with the Los Angeles Raiders. Huizenga says that Rosenfeld had 'one of the largest Beverley Hills practices and took care of a veritable Who's Who of Hollywood stars. But once I stepped into his office, I could see what made him really proud. His walls were plastered with Raider memorabilia and multiple shots of Dr Rosenfeld assisting dazed athletes off the field with thousands of spectators serving as a blurry backdrop' (Huizenga, 1995: 8).

There is, then, an abundance of data which indicates that most sports physicians have an involvement in, and passion for, sport which predates their involvement in the practice of sports medicine. And as we noted in Chapter 5, this passion for sport on the part of the doctor also binds the physician and the patient-athlete together in a distinctive type of doctor-patient relationship, for within this relationship, doctor and patient are bound together not merely by the common medical aim, found in all doctor-patient relationships, of helping the patient to recover, but also by a strong, *extra-medical* consideration: a shared love of sport and, more particularly, a quest for sporting excellence. This is of central importance in understanding the relationship between doctor and patient within sport.

As Freidson has noted, there is often a marked discrepancy between the professional culture of doctors and the lay culture of their patients; however, in the case of the practice of sports medicine – and in marked contradistinction to practice in almost every other branch of medicine – it may be suggested that this gap is largely bridged by the fact that the sports physician shares – one might almost say is *required* to share – the lay sporting culture of their clientele. As Malcolm (2017: 119–120) has noted, the relationship between doctor and their athlete-patient:

> entails clashes between (crudely defined) scientific and lay bodies of knowledge. Stripped of the institutional buttresses that have characterized most of their professional lives, sports medicine clinicians are positioned as outsiders in this cultural milieu (relative to the coaches and athletes who might be defined as the established) and are vulnerable to the influence of their 'less scientific' but more socially powerful, clients.

As we noted in Chapter 5, this situation requires practitioners of sports medicine to commit to two rather different codes of ethics: medical ethics and the lay culture of their athlete-patients, that is the 'sport ethic'. What, then, are the key elements of this 'sport ethic'?

The 'sport ethic' vs medical ethics

Coakley (2009: 163–165) has described the 'sport ethic' as being characterised by the following key values: a dedication to 'the game' above all else, that is to say, the game takes top priority in their lives; a relentless striving for improved performance with a focus on winning and record breaking; an acceptance of risk and a willingness to play through pain and injury; and an unwillingness to accept obstacles in the pursuit of sporting success. Coakley developed the concept of the 'sport ethic' in order to understand the behaviour of elite athletes and, in particular, to understand deviant behaviour such as violence and drug taking. In this regard, Coakley suggests that many forms of deviance within sport may be understood as arising not from a rejection of the norms of the sport ethic, but, on the contrary, as a result of overconformity – that is, an unquestioned acceptance of, and extreme conformity to, these norms in the pursuit of sporting success. Coakley suggests that overconformity is common in elite sport – indeed, he suggests overconformity 'is expected in many sports' – and that 'when athletes don't critically assess the norms of the sport ethic and make a decision to set limits on their conformity, they reproduce a culture in which deviance is common and dangerous'. He adds that this is 'relatively easy to do because people with power in sports pay little attention to overconformity or efforts to control it; instead, they focus on controlling deviant underconformity, such as failing to obey a coach' (Coakley, 2009: 165); a good example of the control of underconformity would be when a player who is not prepared to continue playing through pain and injury may be stigmatised as not being a 'good professional', not having 'the right attitude', or as a malinger (Roderick, Waddington and Parker, 2000: 169). This type of 'overdoing-it deviance', Coakley suggests, involves an overcommitment to the goals of sporting success that may lead, for example, to the willingness to risk serious damage to one's health in order to continue competing and to an acceptance of drug use or other unfair means if these enhance the likelihood of sporting success.

While Coakley's concept of overconformity to the sport ethic was offered as way of understanding aspects of the behaviour of athletes, it is also helpful in understanding those aspects of the behaviour of sports physicians who deviate from what is generally considered good medical practice. In this regard, it may be useful to reiterate some of our key findings concerning sports physicians and the practice of sports medicine. Many sports physicians, as we have seen, have a long-standing and personal commitment to, and passion for, sport; indeed, their love of sport is the major reason why most of them have chosen to work with elite athletes. And we have also seen that, from the early years of the twentieth century, sports medicine not only abandoned the early interest in public health issues, and focused increasingly on elite sport, but that it quickly went beyond a focus on simply treating injuries, as sports physicians became increasingly committed to enhancing the performances of athletes in their charge; indeed, performance enhancement soon became formally recognised as an essential part of the role of the sports doctor. And while their membership of the medical profession requires them to 'buy into' codes of medical ethics, their work situation within elite sport equally requires them to 'buy into' the sport ethic; indeed, it is difficult to imagine how any sports physician could work within elite sport if they were unwilling to accept the principles of the sport ethic. In this sense, it might be said that acceptance of the sport ethic is a precondition for doctors working within elite sport. However, balancing the requirements of the sport ethic with the requirements of medical ethics involves an inherently unstable balance because these two very different codes of ethics – one lay and one professional – involve elements which are not readily compatible: the values associated with health and healing, as opposed to the values associated with performance and winning.

How, then, does an understanding of the dynamic between the sport ethic and medical ethics help us to explain medical involvement in serious unprofessional or deviant behaviour, or malpractice? Put succinctly, why do doctors dope athletes?

Hoberman (2002: 207) has noted that 'a significant number of physicians are motivated by a desire to associate with elite athletes' but he goes on to suggest that this 'may encourage the suspension of professional judgement'. What aspects of the relationship between doctors and athletes might lead to this 'suspension of professional judgement'? We would suggest that a critical aspect of this relationship – in terms of understanding the suspension of professional judgement – is that doctors are likely to identify with the work and success of their athlete-patients to a much greater degree than is the case with their 'ordinary' patients.

In this regard, the relationship between sports physicians and their athlete-patients is very different from the 'normal' doctor-patient relationship in some key respects. Firstly, the doctor and 'patient' within sport are united by the strong shared belief in a set of non-medical values centring on their shared belief in the value of sport and of enhancing performance in the pursuit of sporting excellence; in marked contrast, in most other medical situations the relationship between doctor and patient is unlikely to be premised on anything other than the values of medical science, that is a system of professional health-related beliefs. Secondly, the interaction between doctors and their athlete-patients will normally be far more frequent, and more intense, than the interaction between doctor and patient in other situations. For example, the average patient in the UK visits their general practitioner about three times per year (IDS Media, 2024) with the average consultation lasting ten minutes, so the total interaction time is, on average, about 30 minutes per year. In marked contrast, sports physicians will often work very closely with their athlete-patients and will see them on a frequent and continuing basis, certainly throughout the competitive season, which in many sports extends to nine months of the year. It is also important to stress that in many cases these interactions are not limited to the treatment of injuries – though even these are likely to involve frequent consultations since it will be recalled from the previous chapter that injuries in elite sport are very frequent – but doctors may also be involved, as we have seen, in developing, implementing and monitoring the training programmes of athletes with a view to improving performance. One consequence is that, unlike most general practitioners, who may have difficulty recalling their patients from one consultation to another, the sports physicians and their athlete-patients are likely to develop a close, personal relationship based around the athletes' central goal of sporting success.

Given this close relationship, many sports physicians will become intimately familiar with the goals, aspirations and dreams of the athletes in their charge. And given their own strong and pre-existing commitment to the goal of sporting success, doctors may well come to share those hopes and dreams, and to see themselves as involved in a joint programme, together with their athletes, aimed at securing success. And just as some athletes develop an over-conformity to the sport ethic, so too, it is suggested, do some doctors. Thus while sports physicians have a dual allegiance to medical ethics and to the sport ethic, in some situations their work situation may constrain them to be more responsive to the latter at the expense of the former; in short, the work situation of some sports physicians may constrain them to 'buy into' the sport ethic and to the key goal of sporting success and, at least to some extent, to 'buy out of' medical ethics. In her study of clinicians tasked with the healthcare of Canadian Olympic athletes, Theberge (2007) noted that clinicians learn that their athlete patients principally evaluate health in terms of criteria defined by their athletic performance, while performance was widely seen as the 'default position with regard to the purpose of sports medicine'. Hoberman's (2002: 206) description of physician involvement in the doping process as 'client-centred doping' nicely draws attention to this central aspect of the relationship between 'doping doctors' and their athlete 'patients': their mutual focus on the goal of sporting success.

Jörg Jaksche, a professional cyclist who admitted using drugs while at Team Telekom, said of the two team doctors who were involved in doping riders that: 'I think they were most of all concerned about being close to the athletes and sharing in their success' and he described this as 'A kind of love, a sick sort of affection' (Hacke, 2011). Detlief Hacke, a journalist at *Der Spiegel* who investigated the doping scandal at Team Telekom, had met one of the team doctors, Lothar Heinrich, on several occasions and he reports that Heinrich 'did not view his work as just some job that had to be done. He enjoyed being part of a winning team; he relished the attention, the interviews. He loved to sit on a racing bike' (Hacke, 2011). The comments of Jaksche and Hacke both hint very strongly at an overidentification with the riders and the team and with the overcommitment to their success suggested by Coakley's concept of 'overdoing it deviance'.

Physician behaviour and deviant medical careers: some final thoughts

We have suggested that forms of deviant/unethical behaviour by sports physicians, including their involvement in providing drugs and monitoring their use by athletes, cannot be explained in terms of the individual personality characteristics of sports physicians, but can only be understood by reference to the work situation of practitioners of sports medicine and how this differs from the work situation of doctors in other forms of medical practice. In this regard, we drew attention to the fact that the work situation of many sports physicians means that they may be placed in a situation where they are faced with a conflict of loyalties between the club or sports organisation which employs them and the individual athlete-as-patient. And notwithstanding the fact that although the ethical rules relating to such situations are clear – whatever their contractual obligations, the doctor's primary responsibility is to the individual athlete-as-patient – it is important to recognise that team physicians may come under strong pressure by powerful laypeople within the sportsnet to deviate from the principles of good medical practice, both technically and ethically.

Specifically in relation to drug use, we also emphasised two other critically important characteristics of what, we suggested, was the unique nature of the relationship between doctors and their athlete clients: (i) the fact that the doctor and the athlete are united by a strong mutual commitment to the lay value of sporting success and (ii) that they are likely to have a close relationship such that the doctor comes to share many of the goals of their athlete clients, and that this may lead some doctors, as it undoubtedly leads many athletes, to overcommit to the values of the sport ethic.

But are there any other aspects of the role of the sports physician which might help explain medical involvement in doping? We set out below what might be considered perhaps as some plausible hypotheses, or perhaps as a series of questions for further research.

Within the sociological literature on doctor-patient relationships, a good deal of stress has been placed on the relative power and status of the two parties. In addition to Freidson's work on the significance of the practice location, most emphasis has been placed on the social class and gender dimensions of the relationship between doctors and patients (it will be recalled that in Chapters 1 and 2 we examined the importance of the relative class and status positions of doctor and patient for understanding the practice of medicine in the late eighteenth and nineteenth centuries). In this context, one might ask how the relationship between doctor and athlete is affected by the fact that, while the doctor may occupy a relatively modest place within the medical profession – sports medicine is, after all, hardly the most long-established, or the most prestigious, or the most well paid specialist branch of practice within medicine – their 'patients' may be very wealthy and world famous athletes. In addition, many doctors who work with elite athletes will undoubtedly – and very understandably – derive considerable status, pride and a positive self-image from their association with famous athletes. Once again, this is a distinctive characteristic of sport medicine, for in 'normal' medical practice, doctors do not generally derive any significant status or other social/psychological benefits of this kind from their association with a particular group of patients. Given this unusual aspect of the doctor-patient relationship in elite sport, one might ask whether the dependence of doctors on famous sporting clients for these important social and psychological benefits might mean that the doctor has less power in the relationship with elite athletes than is normally the case in relationships between doctors and their patients.

One might also ask to what extent are physicians, like their athlete clients, constrained by a sporting culture in which greatly increased importance has come to be attached to winning and by a sporting agenda in which 'second place doesn't count'? To what extent do they experience pressure, perhaps not just from the athletes but also from coaches, managers and others, to supply athletes with performance-enhancing drugs? How easy is it to resist such pressures where the prescription of drugs may make the difference between winning and losing an important competition which may involve considerable international prestige? To what extent do doctors themselves understandably wish to be part of a medal-winning or record-breaking team? And is not their participation in a winning team in itself testimony to their professional skill, even if this is used in a way that might generally be considered as deviant?

It is important to note that such a deviant career structure within sports medicine has for many years been firmly established. The Dubin Commission in Canada, for example, noted that Ben Johnson's physician, Dr Jamie Astaphan, 'made an intensive study of anabolic steroids as performance enhancing drugs' and that he became 'very knowledgeable about the various anabolic steroids available through normal suppliers and the black market'. As a result Astaphan developed an international reputation which meant that, in addition to Canadian athletes, he was consulted by athletes from Italy, Holland, Australia, Sweden,

Finland, West Germany, Bulgaria, Jamaica, East Germany, the UK and several African nations (Dubin, 1990: 250–251). Needless to say, the international reputation which he enjoyed was based, as in all client-centred forms of practice, on the lay evaluations of his clients rather than the professional evaluations of his medical colleagues.

It is also clear that doping can be a substantial source of income for practitioners who build up a large practice among athletes; the turnover of Dr Fuente's blood-boosting network in Madrid was estimated to have exceeded 8 million euros in the previous four years (*The Guardian*, 4 July 2006). And the US Anti-Doping Agency (USADA: 2012: 99), recorded that Dr Michelle Ferrari (whose career in doping was described in Chapter 6) received over one million dollars from Lance Armstrong alone and, given that Ferrari worked with very many other elite cyclists over very many years, his total income from doping must have been very substantial indeed. Thus while many forms of practice of sports medicine may offer only very modest rewards, very much larger incomes may be available to those who develop deviant medical careers.

Finally, both authors have, over many years, sought to stress that it is important not to see the drug-using athlete as an isolated individual (Waddington, 2000; Waddington and Smith, 2009; Brissonneau and Montez de Oca, 2018); in exactly the same way it is important not to see drug-prescribing doctors as isolated individuals, but to examine the everyday constraints on their behaviour and the ways in which these constraints might open up deviant careers within medicine.

References

Anderson, L. (2009), Writing a new code of ethics for sports physicians: principles and challenges, *British Journal of Sports Medicine*, 43 (13), 1079–1082.

Anderson, L. and Gerrard, D. F. (2005), Ethical issues concerning New Zealand sports doctors, *Journal of Medical Ethics*, 32, 88–92.

Anderson, L. and Jackson, S. (2013), Competing loyalties in sports medicine: threats to medical professionalism in elite commercial sport. *International Review for the Sociology of Sport*, 48 (2), 238–256.

Brissonneau, C. and Montez de Oca, J. (2018), *Doping in Elite Sports: Voices of French Sportspeople and their Doctors, 1950–2010*. London, Routledge.

British Medical Association (2002), *Drugs in Sport : The Pressure to Perform*, London, BMA.

British Medical Association (2003), *Medical Ethics Today: The BMA's Handbook of Ethics and Law,* London, BMJ Books.

Coakley, J. (2009), *Sport in Society: Issues and Controversies*, tenth edition, Boston, McGraw Hill.

Crane, J. (1990), Association football: the team doctor, in S. D. W. Payne (ed.), *Medicine, Sport and the Law*, Oxford, Blackwell, 331–337.

Devitt, B. M. and McCarthy, C. (2010), 'I am in blood stepp'ed in so far …': ethical dilemmas and the sports team doctor, *British Journal of Sports Medicine*, 44, 175–178.

Dubin, The Hon Charles L. (1990), *Commission of Inquiry into the Use of Drugs and Banned Practices Intended to Increase Athletic Performance*, Ottawa, Canadian Government Publishing Centre.

Faculty of Occupational Medicine (1999), *Guidance on Ethics for Occupational Physicians*, London, Faculty of Occupational Medicine.

Faulkner, A., McNamee, M., Coveney, C. and Gabe, J. (2017), Where biomedicalisation and majic meet: therapeutic innovations of elite sports injury in British professional football and cycling, *Social Science and Medicine*, 178, 136–143.

FIMS (2023), www.fims.org (accessed 7 June 2023).

FIMS (2024) Ethics in sports medicine, *www.fims.org/*. Accessed 17 June 2024.

Freidson, E. (1960), Client control and medical practice, *American Sociological Review*, 65, 374–382.

Freidson, E. (1970), *Profession of Medicine: A Study of the Sociology of Applied Knowledge*, New York, Dodd, Mead.

General Medical Council (1995), *Confidentiality*, London, GMC.

Hacke, D. (2011), From festina to team telekom/team T-mobile. Paper presented to an international symposium, Sportmedizin und Doping in Europa, Evaluierungskommission Freiburger Sportmedizin, University of Freiburg, 12–14 September.

Hoberman, J. (2002), Sports physicians and the doping crisis in elite sport, *Clinical Journal of Sports Medicine,* 12, 203–208.

Hoberman, J. (2012), Sports physicians and doping; medical ethics and elite performance, in D. Malcolm and P. Safai (eds), *The Social Organization of Sports Medicine*, London, Routledge, 237–264.

Holm, S., McNamee, M. and Pi Gozzi, F. (2011), Ethical practice and sports physician protection: a proposal, *British Journal of Sports Medicine*, 45 (15), 1170–1173.

Huizenga, R. (1995), *You're Okay, It's Just a Bruise*, New York, St Martins Griffin.

IDS Media (2024), Who are frequent attenders in primary care? idsmedia.co.uk/news/who-a re-frequent-attenders-in-primary-care, accessed 7 October 2024.

Kennedy, K. W. (1990), The team doctor in rugby union football, in S. D. W. Payne (ed.), *Medicine. Sport and the Law*, Oxford, Blackwell, 315–323.

Lancet (1988), Sports medicine – is there lack of control? *The Lancet*, 2, 612.

Malcolm, D. (2006a), Unprofessional practice? The status and power of sports physicians, *Sociology of Sport Journal*, 23 (4), 376–395.

Malcolm, D. (2006b), Sports medicine: A very peculiar practice? Doctors and physiotherapists in elite English rugby union, in S. Loland, B. Skirstad and I. Waddington (eds.), *Pain and Injury in Sport: Social and Ethical Analysis*, London, Routledge, 165–181.

Malcolm, D. (2009), Medical uncertainty and clinician-athlete relations: the management of concussion injuries in rugby union, *Sociology of Sport Journal*, 26, 191–210.

Malcolm, D. (2014), Sports medicien goes under the knife: The dissection of athlete care, in A. Smith and I. Waddington (eds), *Doing Real World Research in Sports Studies*, London, Routledge, 26–30.

Malcolm, D. (2017), *Sport, Medicine and Health,* London, Routledge.

Malcolm, D., and Scott, A. (2014), Practical responses to confidentiality dilemmas in elite sport medicine, *British Journal of Sports Medicine*, 48 (19), 1410–1413.

Marshall, S. W. and Spencer, R. J. (2001), Concussion in rugby: the hidden epidemic, *Journal of Athletic Training*, 36 (3), 334–338.

McNamee, M., Coveney, C. M., Faulkner, A. and Gabe, J. (2018), Ethics, evidence based sports medicine, and the use of platelet rich plasma in the English Premier League, *Health Care Analysis*, 26 (4), 344–361.

Mitten, M. J. (2002), Emerging legal issues in sports medicine: a synthesis, summary and analysis, *St John's Law Review*, 76 (5), 5–86.

Nixon, H. L. II (1992), A social network analysis of influences on athletes to play with pain and injuries, *Journal of Sport and Social Issues*, 2, 127–135.

Nixon, H. L. II (1993), Accepting the risks of pain and injury in sport: mediated cultural influences on playing hurt, *Sociology of Sport Journal*, 10, 183–196.

Nixon, H. L. II (1994), Coaches vies of risk, pain and injury in sport, with special reference to gender differences, *Sociology of Sport Journal*, 11, 79–87.

Roderick, M., Waddington, I. and Parker, G. (2000), Playing hurt: managing injuries in English professional football, *International Review for the Sociology of Sport*, 35 (2), 165–180.
Roy, S. and Irvin, R. (1983), *Sports Medicine: Prevention, Evaluation, Management and Rehabilitation*, Englewood Cliffs, NJ, Prentice Hall.
Safai, P. (2003), Healing the body in the 'culture of risk': examining the negotiation of treatment between sport medicine clinicians and injured athletes in Canadian intercollegiate sport, *Sociology of Sport Journal*, 20, 127–146.
Scott, A. and Malcolm, D. (2015), 'Involved in every step': how working practices shape te influence of physiotherapists in elite sport, *Qualitative Research in Sport, Exercise and Health*, 7 (4), 539–556.
Theberge, N. (2007), 'It's not about health, it's about performance'. Sport medicine, health and the culture of risk in Canadian sport, in J. Hargreaves and P. Vertinsky (eds), *Physical Culture, Power and the Body*, London, Routledge, 176–194.
United States Anti-Doping Agency (USADA) (2012), *Reasoned Decision of the United States Anti-Doping Agency on Disqualification and Ineligibility*, Colorado Springs, USADA.
Viaud, B. (2009a), Médicines du sport, sports de médicins: quand les biographies sportives s'invitent dans le jeu des carrières professionelles, *Sciences Sociales et Sport*, 1 (2), 129–169.
Viaud, B. (2009b), *Panser les deux mondes. Médecines et sports, entre principes hippocratiques et performances*, PhD Dissertation, Université de Nantes.
Waddington, I. (2000), *Sport, Health and Drugs*, London, Spon.
Waddington, I. (2006), Ethical problems in the medical management of sports injuries: a case study of English professional football, in S. Loland, B. Skirstad and I. Waddington (eds), *Pain and Injury in Sport: Social and Ethical Analysis*, London, Routledge, 182–199.
Waddington, I. (2012), Sports medicine, client control and the limits of professional autonomy, in D. Malcolm and P. Safai (eds), *The Social Organization of Sports Medicine: Critical Socio-Cultural Perspectives,* New York, Routledge, 204–226.
Waddington, I. (2021), Researching pain and injury in sport, in E. C. J. Pike (ed.), *Research Handbook on Sports and Society*, Cheltenham: Edward Elgar, 321–336.
Waddington, I., Roderick, M. and Parker, G. (1999), *Managing Injuries in Professional Football: A Study of the Roles of the Club Doctor and Physiotherapist*, Leicester, Centre for Research into Sport and Society, University of Leicester.
Waddington, I. and Roderick, M. (2002), Management of medical confidentiality in English professional football clubs: some ethical problems and issues, *British Journal of Sports Medicine*, 36 (2), 118–223.
Waddington, I. and Smith, A. (2009) *An Introduction to Drugs in Sport*, London, Routledge.
Waddington, I., Scott-Bell, A. and Malcolm, D. (2019), The social management of medical ethics in sport: confidentiality in English professional football, *International Review for the Sociology of Sport,* 54 (6), 649–665.
Walk, S. R. (1997), Peers in pain: the experiences of student athletic trainers, Sociology of Sport Journal, 14, 22–56.

Index

FSC
www.fsc.org
MIX
Papier | Fördert gute Waldnutzung
FSC® C083411

Kolibri 360 GmbH
Ferdinand-Jühlke-Straße 7
99095 Erfurt, Deutschland
produktsicherheit@kolibri360.de